How to
Live with
a "Neurotic"
at Home
and at Work

Books by ALBERT ELLIS

HOW TO LIVE WITH A "NEUROTIC"
at Home and at Work

by Albert Ellis

CROWN PUBLISHERS, INC., NEW YORK

Printed in the United States of America
Published simultaneously in Canada by General Publishing Company Limited

Designed by Joseph M. Regina

Library of Congress Cataloging in Publication Data
Ellis, Albert, 1913–
    How to live with a neurotic.

    Bibliography: p.
    1. Neuroses. 2. Rational-emotive psychotherapy.
I. Title. [DNLM: 1. Neuroses—Popular works.
WM170 E47h]
RC530.E5 1975   616.8'5   75–4965
ISBN 0–517–520354

Second Printing, October, 1975

Contents

Introduction to the Revised Edition

Out of sheer writing habit I got ready to start this introduction as follows: "This is the first complete book written in E-prime as well as the first E-primer ever written about self-help." Then I stopped. For, according to E-prime, the phrase "This is the first complete book written in E-prime . . ." rings false. E-prime represents a form of writing that never —ah, never!—employs any form of the verb *to be,* including *is, was, am, are, has been,* and so on. As a mode of writing it owes its development to D. David Bourland, Jr., a follower of the general semanticist Alfred Korzybski.

In his famous book *Science and Sanity,* Korzybski lambastes the " 'is' of identity," claiming that when we state that "A is lazy," this means something quite different from the descriptive statement "A does not get up in the morning" or "A refuses to get up in the morning." For the statement "A is lazy" can mean many things and may represent many different orders of abstraction. It may mean, for example, "A sometimes does not get up in the morning," "A rarely gets up in the morning," "A gets up early in the morning but procrastinates about taking a shower," "A deliberately gets up late in the morning," "A tries hard to get up early in the morning, but against his will falls asleep again," and so on. The statement "A is lazy" seems to mean that A always, under all conditions, does things late or never. But *does* it? Usually, of course, it doesn't. But we continually employ such omnibus-sounding statements. Wrongly!

Following up on Korzybski's teachings, D. David Bourland, Jr., originated E-prime, its name coming from the semantic equation: $E' = E - e$, where E represents all the words of standard English and e represents all the forms of "to be." Korzybski held that when we retain the "is" of identity, "we must somehow copy animals in our nervous processes. Through wrong evaluation we are using the lower centres too much and cannot 'think' properly. We are 'overemotional'; we get easily confused, worried, terrorized, or discouraged; or else we become absolutists, dogmatists." Although Korzybski—ironically!—kept employing various forms of "to be" himself in his writings, he did realize how pernicious they can prove. He strongly stated: "When we live in a *delusional* world, we multiply our worries, fears, and discouragements, and our higher nerve centres, instead of protecting us from over-stimulation, actually multiply the semantic harmful stimuli indefinitely. Under such circumstances 'sanity' is impossible."

Bourland, rigorously avoiding the use of "to be" himself, has pointed out various healthy consequences of adopting E-prime:

1. Certain silly and unanswerable questions vanish. One cannot ask, in E-prime, "What *is* my destiny?" "Who *am* I?" And, as I have said in my talks and writings for many years, one had better not! For how can you answer, "Who *am* I?" Though you can often very sensibly answer "What do I like?" "What thoughts and feelings do I have?" "How would I like to live five years from now?"

2. In E-prime some elegantly misleading abbreviations get eliminated, such as "We know this is the right thing to do." These abbreviations involve the "is" of predication.

3. Some hidden expressors of information and feelings get revealed. Instead of "It has been found that," we tend to have "Jones, in his study of polar bears, found that . . ." Instead of "That's where it's at," we can have "I believe your calling Smith a skunk will lead to Smith's firing you." Instead of "Business is business," we can more accurately look for "In the kind of business that I run here, I insist that you stop fooling around and tend to the business itself; else I shall penalize you."

4. The use of E-prime tends to help us expand our awareness of our *linguistic* environment and find means for improving conditions in that environment.

5. With E-prime the degree of completeness, finality, and time independence stated or implied in the verb "to be" vanishes. The "is" of predication leads to such inanities as "Roses are red," which strongly implies that all roses at all times have to remain red.

6. E-prime eliminates absolutistic, self-fulfilling prophecies, especially those of a destructive nature. "I am a success" implies that (1) I have succeeded outstandingly, (2) I will always succeed, and (3) I emerge as a noble, totally good person for succeeding. The first of these statements may well prove false; and the second and the third remain quite unverifiable. The third statement largely consists of a theological, unempirical proposition. "I am a failure" implies (1) I have always failed, (2) I will only and always fail, and (3) the universe has a horror of my failing and will consequently inevitably punish and damn me, and preferably roast me in hell for an eternity, for failing. None of these statements has a good probability of truth, and the last one almost certainly consists of nonsense.

As you can easily see, E-prime has great possibilities in terms of helping humans think straightly about themselves and the world and thereby act more sanely and less neurotically. Some clinical proof of this hypothesis got demonstrated in March 1935, at the First American Congress for General Semantics in Ellensburg, Washington. Dr. John G. Lynn, of McLean Hospital, Waverly, Massachusetts, presented a paper, "Preliminary Report of Two Cases of Psychopathic Personality with Chronic Alcoholism Treated by the Korzybski Method," in which he showed how he had taught Korzybski's Structural Differential method to two seriously disturbed individuals and helped them, within a period of months, to improve significantly.

Since Dr. Lynn's pioneering report, a number of other therapists, including Wendell Johnson, Maxie C. Maultsby, Jr., and myself, have used general semantic principles with their clients, often with fine results. Particularly in recent years, the form of therapy that I originated and developed, rational-emotive therapy (RET), has heavily emphasized many semantic teachings. Consequently, Dr. Donald Meichenbaum and other writers have called it a form of "semantic therapy." Some of the main teachings commonly stressed in RET include:

•interrupting clients when they say "I *must* do this" or "You *should* not do that!" with "Don't you mean '*it would prove better if* you did this'" or "'*it would seem preferable if* you did that'?"

•helping clients change "I can't" to "I won't" and "It's impossible" to "I find it very difficult but *not* necessarily impossible."

•getting people to give up "I *always* feel this way *every* time I do badly at that thing" and say "I *sometimes* feel this way *some of the time* when I do badly at that thing."

•inducing clients to stop thinking and feeling "It is

awful when that *terrible* thing happens" and to think and feel instead "I find it highly inconvenient and disadvantageous when that obnoxious thing happens."

•showing women and men that "It appears bad" rings much truer and brings far better results than "*I* am a *bad person* for doing that bad thing."

•demonstrating to clients that, as Korzybski pointed out in *Science and Sanity,* "We are animals" has nothing to do with the actual facts and implies that we can do nothing about this. But the descriptive phrase "We copy animals in our nervous reactions" may truly describe how we act and makes our "hopeless" behavior turn "hopeful."

•continually combating ethnic, national, and human prejudice by getting people to change their beliefs from "He is a rotten Jew, or a terrible American, or a murderous black" to "He exists as a person who got reared as a Jew and acts rottenly, or who grew up in America and acts very badly, or who got born and raised as a black and behaves murderously."

•showing clients that they do not *need* what they *want, must* not have what they *desire,* can *stand* what they do not *like.*

•teaching people to change their "I'm *supposed to* behave morally" to "*It would most likely prove good* if I behaved morally, because I would get better results if I did," and to change their "Thou *shalt* not steal" to "*It would usually turn out highly preferable* if you did not steal, once you decide to remain a member of a social group, since you would not want others to steal from you, and you would tend to get into serious trouble if you did keep stealing."

•showing clients that their *demands, commands,* and *insistences* usually bring about self-sabotaging results while their *wishes, preferences,* and *desires* bring about better results.

•demonstrating to people that no one *makes* them anxious, depressed, or angry, but that they *make themselves* have or *choose to have* these feelings in their guts.

•helping clients see that statements like "I'm OK, you're OK," or "I like myself," or "I am my own best friend" turn out vague, inaccurate, and misleading. Rather, they'd better say to themselves: "I choose to accept myself and continue to enjoy myself even though I make errors and to accept you and your 'right' to exist and remain happy even though you will continue to do wrong things." And: "I exist and choose to continue to exist and to avoid needless pain and to seek pleasure." And: "I decide to put myself first and others second to myself, just because I decide to do so and think that will bring me better results."

•showing people that because they have often or always failed at something hardly proves that they must keep failing at it.

•proving to clients that their beliefs that "I *must* or *have to* impress others" had best get changed to "It may prove *better* for me to impress others, but I clearly don't *have to* do so, and can remain distinctly happy even if I do not!"

•helping clients and others to understand that "I *become* upset" or that "Others upset me" represent wrong propositions. Instead, "I make *myself* upset by taking events and people *too* seriously."

In these and various other ways RET stresses a semantic approach. In fact, I have hypothesized for the past several years that if some experimenter would train a group of people to use only proper semantic usage, such as Korzybski's Structural Differential, and teach all these individuals to avoid the "is" of identity and all the other forms of overgeneralization that Korzybski and his followers have pointed out, this group actually would turn out "saner," "more rational," and less emotionally "disturbed" than a control group that would not receive this kind of training. A study to test this hypothesis would appear most interesting!

In any event, the time has arrived for me to do something more specific to help bring about the results Korzybski called for: the minimization of our use of the "is" of identity. Accordingly, I have completely revised this edition of *How to Live with a "Neurotic"* in E-prime in the hope that it will make a contribution toward such a goal. Not that it must. Korzybski's and my hypothesis remains nothing but that: a hypothesis. Until someone tests it, no one will really know much about its validity.

I would probably not have gotten around to this move, at least at the present time, had I not had the encouragement and invaluable help of Robert H. Moore, a staff member of the Florida Branch of the Institute for Rational Living, Inc., at Clearwater. Bob, who turned a dedicated E-primist several years ago, has kept urging me (in E-prime, of course!) to get around to this revision; has sent me relevant material on the "is" of identity; and has gone over, at least twice, every word of this revision. Without his help, I doubt that I would have accomplished it.

Not that we haven't had our own differences. We have! As a newly converted purist to E-prime, I at first started revising *How to Live with a "Neurotic"* in a purist or extremist manner. If I originally wrote "A is a neurotic" I changed it to "A has neurotic traits." Or else I made it "We can call A a 'neurotic,'" but put the term "neurotic" in quotation marks to make it clear that I realize, as the writer of this term, that we cannot accurately label A as *a* "neurotic," since we then imply that he *always* and *only*, for all time, can act neurotically. Hence the compromise use of quotations around the word "neurotic."

Technically I remain correct, and even go Korzybski and, at times, Bourland one better, since they accept the looser terminology "We can call A a neurotic," and thereby get rid of the "is" but keep the implication that we can thereby label A accurately. We can't! The essence of Korzybski's philosophy holds that all things change. A rose, therefore, "is" not red, because it may later turn black or some other color. It "is" not even a rose, since it may turn to dust or to other elements. Similarly, A "is" not a "neurotic," because his neurosis may change: vanish, improve, or get worse. But to say, as Korzybski and Bourland might say in E-prime, "I classify A as a neurotic" or "I see A as a neurotic" still proves incorrect, at least technically. Still too general: still too inclusive! We might say something like "I classify A as a neurotic at this particular moment in time, knowing that he doesn't act completely neurotically but mainly so, and that he may well change his neurotic behavior and wind up as less neurotic or non-neurotic in the future."

Such a formulation, however, seems quite awkward and requires us to make practically every statement about A in a highly qualified, long-winded manner. Accurate, perhaps— but how practical? After discussing this matter with Bob Moore, I let his arguments (and the usage of Korzybski and Bourland) at least partly prevail. In this revision I don't remain purist and do use terms like "a disturbed individual" and "a helper," although I know they come off as partial overgeneralizations. Though I place the term "neurotic" in quotation marks—to emphasize the fact that I really don't believe that anyone only or always possesses "neurotic" behavior or traits—I don't bother to keep putting a "disturbed individual" or a "helper" in quotation marks as well. Perhaps, in some of my future writings, I shall return to a purist position and either avoid using terms like these at all or else consistently put them in quotation marks. But not in the present revision!

Also, although this at times may seem confusing, I only

put the word "neurotic" in quotation marks in this book when I use it as a noun. When I say "He has neurotic behavior" or "She acts neurotically," I do not use special quotation marks, but when I say "She acts like a 'neurotic'" or "'Neurotics' often behave badly," I do put "neurotic" in quotes. Why? Because although "He has neurotic behavior" constitutes a mild overgeneralization (actually he *sometimes* under *certain* conditions has this behavior), "She acts like a 'neurotic'" constitutes a stronger overgeneralization (as it implies that she *always* and *only* acts neurotically and that such an entity as a thoroughly neurotic *person* actually exists). So, to reiterate, I keep the term "neurotic" as an adjective or adverb without putting it in quotation marks, but when I use the term "neurotic" as a noun I put it in quotation marks.

Semantic and linguistic revisions alone do not make up this new edition of *How to Live with a "Neurotic."* I intended to revise the book completely, anyway, since the system of rational-emotive therapy that I described in the first edition has developed considerably since I originated it in 1955 and described it in some detail in 1957. Some of the newer concepts of RET now presented in this book include:

Non-absolutistic thinking. I have come to realize more than ever, over the years, that while exaggerated thinking ("I'd better get perfect marks to get through school") creates some degree of emotional disturbance, absolutistic thinking ("I *must* get perfect marks to get through school") proves even more pernicious and lies at the roots of more serious and pervasive disturbance. Consequently, RET therapists (such as those we train at our clinic at the Institute for Advanced Study in Rational Psychotherapy in New York City) learn to zero in quickly on any stated or implied absolutes—shoulds, oughts, musts, necessities—that people use to disturb themselves, and to teach their clients to dispute, actively and vigorously, these musts. Where, in the first edition of this book, I used such phrases as "one must withdraw emotion-ally" from a "neurotic" individual who refuses to change, I now point out that "one had better withdraw emotionally" from such an individual—but one doesn't *have* to.

Individual worth. As I indicated in more detail in my later books (such as *Growth through Reason, The Sensuous Person,* and *Humanistic Psychotherapy: The Rational-Emotive Approach*), as well as in the revised edition of *A Guide to Rational Living* (written with Dr. Robert A. Harper), I have changed my previous stand that people have intrinsic worth or value and that they can legitimately say, "I exist as good because I remain alive." I now believe that we cannot legitimately rate a total human as either good or bad, that intrinsic value proves a rather meaningless and un-definable term, and that we would achieve better, less dis-turbed results if humans did not evaluate themselves, their essences, at all.

Homework. More than ever, over the years, RET has developed the concept of activity and thinking homework assignments: of inducing people who want to change their thinking and their disordered emoting to work and practice against their present states, both in their heads and in their actual lives. When I created RET, behavior therapy prac-tically did not exist, and RET first clearly stated some of its outstanding theories and practices. It persuaded clients to *act* against their fears, to *practice* new kinds of thinking, to de-liberately *stay* in obnoxious situations at times in order to show themselves that they could *stand* such situations. It also employed techniques of self-management (or what B. F. Skinner calls operant conditioning): using rewards or rein-forcements when they did the sensible thing and penalties when they did the self-defeating thing. Since the early days of RET, I and my associates (including Dr. H. Jon Geis, Dr. William Knaus, Edward Garcia, and Dr. Maxie C. Maultsby,

Jr.) have developed homework assignments and systematized them. Some of this new emphasis gets included in the present revision.

Blaming and damning. From the start RET has stressed the importance of people's refraining from blaming themselves (and others) for their poor performances. It still does! But linguistically, if I tell you "Don't blame yourself for making an error," you can easily think I mean "Don't admit that you made an error; or admit it, but don't take it at all seriously, nor do much to correct it." I mean, of course, "By all means acknowledge fully that you have made this error; realize how handicapping it proves; and work like hell to minimize or eliminate it in the future. But don't, under any conditions, excoriate *yourself* for making it. Don't *damn* or *vilify* yourself in any way for acting erroneously. Don't *down* yourself!" To make this point clearer, I make little use of the word "blame" in this revision, but instead keep using "damn," "down," and equivalent terms.

Inappropriate and appropriate emotions. When I wrote the first edition of *How to Live with a "Neurotic,"* I erroneously believed that sadness or unhappiness could legitimately arise, but that if you felt extremely or unduly sad or unhappy, you behaved neurotically. Now I realize that even exceptional sorrow or displeasure may prove appropriate, as long as you have very strong wants or preferences and these keep getting thwarted. I now see illegitimate or inappropriate emotions, such as depression, anxiety, despair, shame, and hostility as usually arising from absolutes; not from your strongly *desiring* that you get what you want but from your *commanding, demanding,* or absolutistically *insisting* that you get it. Thus, if you say "I want A to love me very much," and A does not love you, you can make yourself appropriately sad, sorrowful, regretful, displeased, unhappy, or even miserable. But if you say "I *must* have A love me; I find it *awful* if she or he doesn't; I turn into a *rotten person* if A's love for me vanishes," you make yourself depressed, anxious, despairing, self-downing, and possibly suicidal. In this revised edition I develop the theme of appropriately and inappropriately emoting, and thereby add some new RET developments.

These and several other up-to-date RET concepts get included in the revised edition of *How to Live with a "Neurotic."* For these reasons, as well as the rewriting of the book in E-prime, I think it will prove more useful than ever to large numbers of readers. I have heard, by mail and personal contact, from literally thousands of people who have helped themselves immensely by reading this book. May their numbers now significantly increase!

ALBERT ELLIS, Ph.D.

Institute for Advanced Study in Rational Psychotherapy
New York City

Introduction

One of the most frequent questions asked by my clients and acquaintances goes like this: "Tell me, Dr. Ellis, about what percentage of people in our society would you say act neurotically?" I generally reply: "Roughly, about a hundred."

Do I mean this seriously? Not entirely. From an ideal standpoint, people behave neurotically when, potentially intelligent and capable, they perform stupidly and act self-defeatingly. In this sense, virtually all of us appear more or less "disturbed."

From a more practical standpoint, however, we usually label as "neurotic" those whose feelings seem so inappropriate and whose behavior appears so ineffective or disruptive that they often feel anxious, depressed, hurt, or hostile. In this sense, I would say, as a rough estimate, that between 30 and 50 percent of us frequently behave neurotically.

This means, if I estimate correctly, that millions of people have emotional problems, many of which even the untrained layman can detect. What, if anything, can we do? Assuming that you have only a moderate disturbance yourself, and that some of your associates have more, what can you do to live comfortably with troubled individuals and to try to help them? The present book tries to answer this question.

To illustrate what often happens when one person closely associates with another who has a serious disturbance, consider the cases of two people who happened to consult me on the same afternoon. The first, a woman of thirty, married for six years, had a husband who, while not doing anything else outlandish, had given her no money during this time. He paid the rent and food bills, sat at home reading on those few nights of the week when he did not attend a meeting of one of the numerous organizations to which he belonged, and had intercourse with her about once a month. Otherwise, he did nothing to earn the name of husband. Helping or playing with their two children, taking his wife to a show, telling her about what had happened at the office, discussing with her the latest news—he did none of these things. Yet when I spoke to him, he saw nothing unusual about his marriage, did not understand why his wife felt so unhappy, and sincerely believed that they had a comfortable, fine relationship.

The second client, a fifty-year-old man, married for twenty-nine years, had a wife who, during all this time, had confined herself to their home. She maintained friendly relations only with her mother, had sex about four times a year, and insisted that she made an excellent wife because she never missed cooking a meal or sending the family's dirty clothes to the laundry. This woman, like the husband of my first client, obviously had a serious disturbance. She felt such fear of doing anything outside a very simple, rigid routine that she lived on the narrowest possible plane of existence and had distorted ideas about what constituted a good marriage.

What could both my clients do? I explained to them, when I realized what disturbances their mates had, that they

2

could do one of three things: seek a divorce or separation; encourage their spouses to receive psychological treatment; or continue to live with their untreated mates and learn to put up with their disturbances.

Usually, in cases like this, clients see the first of the three alternatives as undesirable or impractical, since separation or divorce, especially involving children, means heartache and hardship. They see the second alternative as desirable but unfeasible, because the mate will refuse to accept professional treatment. They find living with a "neurotic" and avoiding driving themselves to the brink of despair, the third alternative, both desirable and practical.

To help you try this solution, I have developed a teaching technique that tells you exactly what to do to live successfully with a "neurotic." This book outlines some of the elements of this teaching.

For example, I enabled the thirty-year-old woman to see her husband as an exceptionally frightened and insecure person, who felt he had suffered seriously in his relationships with his mother and two previous woman friends, and consequently felt loath to get emotionally involved with anyone else lest he again experience rejection and feel "destroyed." When his wife understood this, and persisted in giving him warmth and security in spite of his initial coolness, he gradually warmed up, drew considerably closer to her, committed himself to the risks of emotional involvement, and displayed more devotion.

The case of the fifty-year-old man did not get so easily resolved. His wife proved to have a borderline psychosis and barely maintained her hold on reality by living in a highly restricted fashion. She didn't want therapeutic help, and even consistent kindness and devotion by her husband could not unthaw her. I taught him, finally, to accept her with her disturbance and to see that her coldness resulted from

3

this disturbance rather than from his own behavior. He had essentially two choices: to separate from his wife or to accept her *with* her borderline state. Since he did not wish, partly for religious reasons, to take the first choice, I helped him to take the second, to realistically inure himself to the fact that he lived with a frequently disturbed woman.

These two cases typify, not the problems that beset individuals living with "neurotics" or "psychotics," but the choices they confront. For assuming that you live, for whatever reasons, with a consistently disturbed spouse, relative, friend, or business associate, you usually have innumerable bad choices but only two or three good ones. Either you choose to help this person get less disturbed and easier to live with or, if you won't or can't do this, you choose to live with him or her in spite of the continuing disturbance, with a minimum of distress to yourself. In some instances you can use a combination of these two sensible approaches.

In trying to show you how to live successfully with a "neurotic," this book may also give you some valuable insights into yourself and your own "neurotic" trends. For one of the best ways to know yourself comes through understanding and helping others.

Take, by way of illustration, another of my clients. A young mother came to see me because she regularly had serious difficulties with her mother-in-law, who insisted on telling her just how to handle her child, how to treat her husband, and how to manage her life. Having felt rebellious toward her own mother, and having no intention of acquiring an even more dominant overseer through her marriage, she typically fought tooth and nail with her mother-in-law, much to the distress of everyone involved, especially her husband.

I let her do considerable talking, at first, about her mother-in-law. I came to understand that the mother-in-law had the best of intentions—but the worst of anxieties. She

4

would not, in her own life, make even the tiniest decision for fear of making a horrible mistake. She therefore kept trying to make other people's (including her daughter-in-law's) decisions for them. She could thereby evade any responsibility or self-condemnation if, somehow, these decisions turned out wrong, since she had not *actually* made them.

My client began to see that what she previously had considered her mother-in-law's strength and overdecisiveness actually masked this woman's weakness and indecisiveness. Seeing this, she began to lose her antagonism; and, instead of resenting the older woman's attempts to boss her around, she now began to pity her and to try to give her more love and security. Relations between the daughter-in-law and mother-in-law eventually grew almost cordial!

One day the client came to me and spontaneously said: "You know, I've had a chance to think about how my mother-in-law used to act with me and the reasons for her acting as she did. And it occurred to me, as I told my oldest daughter how to do her schoolwork the other day, that I have something of my mother-in-law in me, too. After all, I had a bullying mother, just as she had, and I tended to let my mother have a serious effect on me, too—my indecisiveness, I mean. I often hesitate dreadfully in doing things.

"And as I heard myself tell my daughter how to do her schoolwork the other day, I suddenly got the picture of my mother-in-law doing exactly the same sort of thing to me. I realized for the first time how much we have in common. I don't like contemplating that, naturally. But I sure do see it!

"Would you believe it—when I saw that, I suddenly stopped, right in the middle (the middle, I mean, of telling my daughter about her schoolwork), and I said to myself, 'Now look here—stop bullying that child. You just want her to act better than you do, to behave more decisively. But that way won't work. You'll just continue to avoid, instead of to face, your own problems. Let the child alone! You behave just as badly as your mother-in-law!' And I did stop right there, and told her she could do the work any way she liked, as long as it satisfied her. I felt much better after that."

Understanding others, then, often opens the road to understanding yourself. And understanding others' disturbances halves the battle to understand your own neurotic trends. If we live, as we seem to live, in an age and a culture in which emotional disturbances flourish, we'd better face the fact that we ourselves may well have some degree of disturbance. And, in addition, we go through life encountering and often getting involved with others' hangups.

Can we recognize, understand, and help with some of the neurotic problems with which we keep coming into contact? The fundamental premise of this book holds that we can.

1

The Possibility of Helping Troubled People

To live successfully with, and to help people with problems, you'd better believe that they *can* profit by your help. And they can. For, as humans, we learn (or teach ourselves) our neuroses; and anything we learn, we normally can unlearn.

The "neurotic's" feeling of hopelessness hangs on *belief* in his or her hopelessness. This appears as one of the most distinctive, and, one might say, most human, characteristics of men and women: that what they *believe* in they usually *accept* as truth; what they *think* they can't change, they *can't* change. But if humans believe they *can* change, they almost always can actualize this belief. And if you believe that you can help them change, you have an excellent chance of doing so.

I once saw an outstanding lawyer. After twenty-five years of marriage, he had still not learned to satisfy his wife sexually, and when I suggested some obvious ways, he immediately objected: "But how can I change my sex habits, Dr. Ellis, after having them so long?"

"You," I responded, "regard yourself as a good trial lawyer, do you not?"

belief of hoplessness → feeling of hoplessness.

EG ↓

"Yes, I think so."

"And every time you get a new case, you carefully plan it according to your past experience with this kind of case, and with judges and juries, do you not?"

"Yes, surely."

"Well," I said, "suppose, after working on one of your cases for a while, you discover that your plan doesn't work. What do you do—stubbornly stick to it, because you originally outlined it that way?"

"Why, of course not. I plan a new strategy, make another effort."

"Why, then, don't you do the same thing about sex with your wife? Your old strategy hasn't worked for twenty-five years. What do you plan to do—use it for another twenty-five?"

"I never thought about it that way."

"Well, don't you believe you'd better—assuming that sex with your wife means as much to you as winning a court case?"

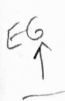

P.S. He did start to think about it and soon worked out a much better adjustment.

People, then, feel hopeless and often look hopeless as long as they think themselves hopeless, and consequently make no effort to change. For change involves effort; and effort involves a goal, an idea. And the essence of change itself derives from the *idea* that things can get better—that they can change. Observe how the concept of hope negates hopelessness.

Applied to the "neurotic" with whom you have steady contact, this means that if you have a concept that he or she may change, an idea that he or she need not remain hopelessly disturbed, you probably have gone halfway toward effectively helping. And I have spent many years as a practicing therapist giving exactly this concept to my clients who intimately associate with troubled people.

Consider one man who consulted me because, while he *E-G* worked at finishing his graduate studies, his wife got exceptionally jealous of his school activities. As soon as he settled down with his books, she would stop her reading or television-viewing, and start talking to him about irrelevant, unimportant things. When he pointed out that he had to study, she said that his work obviously meant more to him than she did, that he never spent any time with her, and that he clearly didn't love her anymore. This led to a lengthy argument, which, by the time they had calmed down, generally consumed the evening, and left his scholastic tasks undone.

At my urging the husband tried a different tack. Before he did any schoolwork, he spent a period of time expressing warmth to his wife, telling her that he loved her, and sometimes making sexual advances. He discussed his school activities with his wife and made an effort to get her to feel as much concern about them as he felt himself. He told her, especially, about his difficulties with this professor or that instructor, and asked her how she thought he could handle these situations.

Finally, my client induced his wife to help him with his lessons. He had her do some of his typing and arithmetic, and read to him when his eyes got tired. She soon took a vital interest in his work and felt she practically belonged in class with him. After a few weeks of this new approach, which succeeded in winning her active cooperation, they began to get along much better. Her neurotic self-downing lessened as she saw herself making a valuable contribution to her husband's education.

The same kind of plan will work with many "neurotics." To try to argue or bully them out of their disturbed behavior frequently makes things worse. But if you attempt to discover why they act the way they do, and what you can do about

don't argue y or bully the neurotic

9

getting them to act better, you have an excellent chance of helping them—and, of course, helping yourself at the same time. For people often act more psychologically than logically. If you treat them in an understanding way, you can accomplish wonders in some of the seemingly most "hopeless" cases.

Understanding and helping others depends largely upon how you see things. Most people get so involved in their own problems and worries that they take little time or energy to comprehend anyone else's point of view. If you can manage to see things from another's vantage point, you can often provide inestimable help.

Relevant here, I recall the case of a woman, an excellent secretary, who normally enjoyed her job. Because she upset herself about her husband's criticism, however, she began doing badly at work, lost her interest in it, and wanted to quit. Her husband opposed this and pointed out that they could well use the money she earned. She tried explaining her feelings, but to no avail. She began to feel guilty, as well as depressed.

As I frequently do in this type of case, I decided to try to use the husband as an auxiliary therapist, and I asked to see him. He spent most of our first session complaining about his wife's "unreasonable" desire to quit work. He thought she did an excellent job for her employer and that she would feel much happier working than not working. He didn't understand why she couldn't see this.

I carefully explained to him that, theoretically, his position made good sense. If his wife left her job, she not only would hate herself for running away when the going got rough, but also would lose the confidence she derived from her competency at work, and might therefore tend to feel more ineffective in other respects. She then might hate herself even more, creating a vicious circle.

10

The husband, gratified to hear that I agreed with his analysis, positively beamed, and indicated that he would now go home and belabor his wife with my words and thereby get her to do things his way. I could vividly see him loading his shotgun with the verbal ammunition I had just supplied.

"You've got the point," I said. "But let's look at the thing another way for a moment. Your wife, by wanting to quit work, acts illogically, against her own best interest. But does *she* see it that way? Does she not, rather, feel that just because she now does poorly on the job, she will lower her confidence by remaining on it, and will then perform worse in other respects? Doesn't this encourage her to feel *forced* into leaving, even though she knows the disadvantages, monetary and otherwise, of doing so?"

Yes, he could see that, he said.

"And let us go one step further," I continued. "Your wife knows that, when she did well on her job a while ago, she still got into trouble with you—about the housework and things like that—doesn't she?"

"Yes, I guess so."

"And now that she contemplates leaving work, she knows how unhappy you feel about this?"

"Yes."

"Well, if—to her way of looking at things—doing a good job doesn't satisfy you and brings her little of the reward she really wants—your love and consideration—why should she keep rewarding you for what gets her beaten over the head? Why would it not make more sense—seeing things, again, from *her* frame of reference—for her to do something that would punish you for the unjust way that she thinks you generally treat her?"

"Now that you put it that way, I guess it might."

"Exactly. So I think you'll understand what you've actually done—even though you haven't realized it. You've

11

punished her when she does well (on the job, for instance) by criticizing her about the housework. Then, when she does poorly, and thinks of quitting, you unconsciously reward her by letting her see how unhappy you feel. From her point of view, therefore, if she wants to get back at you for what she considers your unfair criticism, how might she best do this?"

"Just the way she does it now, I guess—punish me by wanting to quit her job."

"Right. So she really doesn't seem so crazy after all, does she?"

"I should say not!"

By showing this husband how to understand and see things from his wife's frame of reference, I helped him to diminish his criticism of her. He stopped making an issue of her every fault and inadequacy. He minimized some foolish things she did, pretended not to notice others, and generally employed a more constructive approach. Sensing his changed attitude, she began rewarding him—and herself—by doing better at her work, which soon killed any question of her leaving her job.

In this instance I helped a woman with neurotic thinking to remove some of the pressure she put on herself by first having her husband remove *his* pressure. When he began to see her actions in *her* frame of reference and to treat her with understanding, she recognized her own distortions of reality and did something about them. When her husband accepted her as a wife and as a human, she accepted herself as an effective secretary as well.

This did not, of course, represent an ideal solution to her problem. She might have profited more if, in spite of her husband's severe criticism, she had decided to accept herself fully—decided, for instance, that she *wanted* but did not *need* his love, and that she could have distinct (though decreased) enjoyment even though he cared less.

In any event, "neurotics" can learn to see things differently themselves, and hence to change their disturbed behavior. And they learn particularly well when others begin to see them in a different light and to give them leeway to move along less neurotic pathways.

Sometimes still more direct methods help emotionally perturbed people solve their problems. A mother came to see me about her twenty-one-year-old daughter's fear of staying alone in the house. The daughter insisted that one or both of her parents remain with her whenever she stayed at home. I tried to see the daughter, but she refused to come in for even one session. I, therefore, worked through the mother, who served as an auxiliary therapist.

I asked the mother, in this case, to try a planned method of deconditioning the daughter's fears of remaining alone. I got her to visit a nearby neighbor, ostensibly for a few minutes, and then deliberately stay longer. She called from the neighbor's, from time to time, to tell the daughter that for some reason she would delay returning a few minutes longer. Gradually, she built up the time of staying away from ten to twenty minutes, and then increased it to thirty or forty minutes.

Every time the mother stayed away for any length of time, she would remark (on my instructions) as soon as she got in: "Sorry Mrs. So-and-So detained me, but you know how gabby she can get. Anyway, you seem to have done fine in my absence. Why, I've actually stayed away thirty minutes, and you've done beautifully. I always knew you could and I'll bet you don't really feel so afraid anymore." Eventually, after continuing to lengthen her visits over a period of several months, her daughter got more and more used to the idea that she could get along by herself and actually remain alone in the house. She gradually got over her fears.

We find many ways, then, of helping a "neurotic." None

13

of them succeeds with enormous ease; some require considerable effort. But if you take the time and trouble to apply
them, they work—and often work better than your wildest
expectations lead you to believe. Not that you can expect
miracles, although people often describe as miraculous what
happens to a person when a properly coached member of the
family helps him or her emotionally.

Said one of my clients: "I can't thank you for what you
have done for us, for me and my family, Doctor. It seems like
a miracle."

I replied: "Not what *I've* done, but what *you've* done
has accomplished this 'miracle.' I, as I told you during our
very first session, can help you understand things, can point
out ways in which you can aid yourself. But *you* do them, act
on them. I can't do anything for you; you can work—and have
worked—beautifully to help yourself. You really have yourself to thank."

This woman accepted her nineteen-year-old daughter's
harsh verbal attacks, which had continued for almost ten
years. Instead of making herself angry as she had done before
coming to see me, she began to understand how and why
they arose, and to meet them with concern and kindness. The
result, achieved within six weeks, amazed her. The daughter
not only stopped berating the mother, but began cooperating,
desisted from spending all her time in the college library,
and began dating boys. A real "miracle." Yet, only a little
understanding, a changed maternal attitude, occurred. Nothing but that—and a nineteen-year-old who seemed doomed
to self-downing and hostility now had more than an even
chance to enjoy herself and to relate to others.

Can anyone help anyone else to overcome emotional
quirks and upsets? No, not exactly. For the prospective
helper, aside from having good intentions and real patience,

better not have too severe a disturbance; ditto, the helpee. Individuals with severe problems should preferably see professionals; and those who would help them can obtain psychological consultation. Otherwise, more harm than good may result.

This means, specifically: Don't try to cure your friends or relatives who feel exceptionally depressed, who think very little of themselves, who experience unusual agitation, or who behave bizarrely. Such individuals may prove psychotic and require immediate professional care and sometimes institutionalization. By all means try to get them to those with training.

The fact remains, however, that many of our intimates do not require professional care—even though almost all of them might well benefit from at least a few consultations. And many who would better have intensive psychotherapy, simply won't. These people can often get considerable help through the wise intercession of a friend or relative willing to take the time and trouble to understand them and to assist in guiding them through their perplexity.

Instructive in this connection: The case of a mother who came to see me to complain that her twenty-nine-year-old unmarried daughter didn't really care to try to find a husband. She went on dates with males, but somehow didn't go with the marrying kind; and whenever my client pointedly brought this fact to her attention, the daughter would argue and scream like a fishwife and tell her to mind her own business. What, the mother asked, could she do with a child like that?

I, too, tried to get the mother to mind her own business. I attempted to show her that, if her daughter did not marry, she probably just didn't want to. Or, if she did, she perhaps did not have sufficient confidence to try to find the right kind of man; or she disturbed herself so much about her mother's incessant proddings that she possibly enjoyed spiting the mother by not marrying. Anyway, I said, at twenty-nine years, what she did or did not do about marriage fell well beyond her mother's control. The less the mother nagged her, the more likely she would get married.

The mother couldn't see this at all, and thought that I had collaborated somehow with her daughter (and the devil) to keep her unmarried. I saw that I wouldn't get anywhere, since she didn't face her own contribution to the "problem," and kept insisting that I see her daughter as unbalanced and ungrateful. So I asked her to send the daughter to see me. I frankly hadn't thought so much of working with the daughter—though she probably could use the help, too—except to see whether I could induce her to assist me with the mother's problem.

When the daughter came in, I realized immediately that she really had problems. But she acknowledged this willingly and wanted to do something to help herself. After several visits, she developed insight and began to see, as I had guessed from my first talk with the mother, that she resented her mother's prodding her into marriage, and resisted by selecting unmarriageable boyfriends. Putting this insight to good use, she began to get more selective in her choice of steady dates and to work toward a good relationship with one of them.

In the meantime, even before she changed her dating pattern, I got her to help me with the mother's problem. After I explained her parent's disturbance, the daughter stopped arguing with her mother and, at my suggestion, calmly accepted almost everything she said. Realizing her mother's overanxiety, she would tell her mother just what she wanted to hear about the men she, the daughter, dated. No matter how outlandish or provocative the advice, she calmly went—or at least seemed to go—along with whatever her mother said (even though, in practice, she often completely ignored her mother's views).

When the mother, impressed with the daughter's changed attitudes, and especially with her newfound serenity, found nothing negative to respond to, she began to calm down. She came to see me several weeks later, apologized for her previous antagonism, and said that she loved the changes I had wrought in her daughter, who had begun to behave like "a completely different girl."

Actually, the daughter had not changed that much, although she had begun to tackle her own basic problems and eventually (some six months later) solved many of them. The mother, ironically, considerably improved herself. Her daughter's example of determined, reasonable behavior removed much of her own excuse for irrationality. Where I, as psychotherapist, at first failed to make any inroads on the mother's neurosis, the daughter's insight and actions helped enormously.

My intimate association with many cases like these encourages me to believe that, with the proper knowledge and effort, almost any nonprofessional without too many problems can help a close relative, friend, or associate who has more troubles—providing, of course, the helper understands neurosis, its probable causes, and some of the methods that can change neurotic behavior patterns. With this knowledge, and a strong determination to apply it in practice, he or she can often achieve remarkable results.

What, then, does "neurotic" mean, and what makes a person "neurotic"? Let us see.

2

How to Recognize a Person with Emotional Disturbance

Who qualifies as a "neurotic"?

Basically, an adult who consistently acts illogically, irrationally, inappropriately, and childishly.

Although, theoretically they can think for themselves and plan their days for effective, happy living, "neurotics" actually fall back on unintelligent behavior, fail to attain some of their dearest goals, and sabotage their best potentialities.

Will you, then, easily recognize "neurotics" when you meet them?

Not necessarily. For you will find many *truly* stupid people around. These individuals, because of inherited or early acquired mental defects, do not think clearly, act grown-up, do things effectively. They do not have the intelligence to plan and execute rational modes of living. Not knowing enough to come in out of the rain, they frequently get soaking wet. But because there exists a definite physical

18

(neurological) reason for their nonrational, childish behavior, we cannot accurately label them "neurotic."

Neurosis, moreover, may get confused with unhappiness. *≠ unhappn* Some people—millions, in fact—behave *appropriately* unhappily. Take, for instance, those who do not have enough to eat, who work at poor jobs, or who have chronic illness. Can they reek with happiness?

"Neurotics," then, make themselves *unreasonably* or *unnecessarily* bothered or bewildered. They bring on more pain or anxiety than they, theoretically, need experience. Many of them have more than enough wherewithal—good looks, high intelligence, fine talents—to get along successfully in this world. But somehow they don't. That "somehow," that "something," that comes between their potential abilities and their actual achievements—*that* we call "neurosis."

We cannot easily say who acts and who does not act disturbed for the fundamental reason that "neurotics" cover up marvelously. They want, last of all, recognition for their degree of foolishness or neurosis. They resort to all kinds of subterfuges and defenses to prevent recognition of their true emotional colors. They compartmentalize, for instance, and *compartmtlz* hold their neurotic behavior to one or two major aspects of their lives, while acting with reasonable normality in most other respects. Or they compensate and do a splendid job in *compensatn* one area—such as in their business dealings—while virtually falling apart in other respects. Or they go through silly rituals and magical devotions within the confines of their own homes but act convincingly sane on the outside.

Many "neurotics," consequently, seem happy and effective to some of their closest associates, even though a pitiably thin line separates them from serious disturbance.

We have another obstacle in the way of recognizing neurotic symptoms in their almost infinite variety. "Neurotics" tend to act peculiarly—to some degree irrationally

19

and "crazily." But the roads to emotional perplexity remain many. Where one "neurotic" has terrible fears of doing almost anything, another shows his disturbance by needlessly risking his neck every day in some dangerous enterprise. While one lies abed all day and refuses to do any work, another frantically consumes himself in a dozen violent endeavors. One woman insists that she has wasted away from a score of imaginary ills; and another with a cancerous ovary insists that she has no disease, that death does not exist, and that her Yoga breathing exercises will take care of all her ills.

A further problem in distinguishing neurosis from other forms of irregular behavior emerges in the fact that eccentricity and neurosis differ. Virtually all "neurotics" behave, in one way or another, eccentrically; but not all "eccentrics" behave neurotically. If a Henry David Thoreau, for example, wants to desert Concord society for a while to live in the Walden woods, or if a Mahatma Gandhi wishes to lead a movement of passive resistance against the British, these eccentricities and heresies do not necessarily constitute proof of emotional aberration. Rebels and saints occasionally display craziness, but not always.

You can—though not easily—disagree profoundly with the great majority of your fellows and yet, in your own life's goals and ideals, act consistently. Neurosis suggests an *inner* contradiction, a discord between what you want to do for yourself and the means you use to achieve your goals. Eccentricity may merely entail a contradiction between your ideals and those of your neighbors. It does not *have* to, though it may, constitute a symptom of disturbance.

How, in view of some of the confusing evidence and of our inability to see inner contradictions and unconscious conflicts, can we tell a "neurotic" from a so-called "normal" or "well-adjusted" individual? Mainly, by recognizing his or her most important neurotic manifestations or symptoms. Some of the main symptoms of emotional disturbance include: *indecisn*

Indecision, doubt, and conflict. "Neurotics" often act with *doubt* *conflict* indecision, hesitancy, doubt. They want to do something but fear making a mistake, failing in their own and others' eyes. So they waiver, decline to make decisions, refuse to commit themselves or to take full responsibility for almost anything.

One woman I knew left her husband to live with another man, but then kept finding fault with her lover because he lacked some of the characteristics of the husband. She waivered between the two, and literally shuttled back and forth between them several times, before she finally saw that the real issue involved not *their* traits but her *own* indecisiveness. When she faced this fact, and started to work on her own problems, she had no trouble making up her mind—in this instance in favor of the husband.

Fear and anxiety. Virtually all "neurotics" have an irrational fear of something. On the surface they may appear the *fear &* *anxiety* fearless, mountain-climbing type. Underneath—jelly. More than anything else they fear what people think—feel terrified of not having others love and approve of them. Sometimes they honestly admit this. But often they translate their fears of disapproval into more concrete phobias, such as the fear of walking on the street, or of staying cooped up at home. Look beneath their defenses and you'll find an irrational dread.

What gives "neurotics" the shakes? Everything imaginable! I have seen strong, hulky brutes of men who have quailed at the sight of a small bug, or who refused to take a plane trip, or who broke into a sweat at the mere idea of going to a party, or who would not go through with a job interview if their lives depended on it. I have seen women who bore five children without flinching who would go into an extreme state of panic at the contemplation of exchanging an article in a store, or of getting examined by a physician, or of eating a

21

banana, or of giving a bridge party. Some of the physically bravest "neurotics" feel terribly afraid of what others may say or think.

Inadequacy feelings. People with emotional problems often feel inadequate, worthless, or wicked. They think that they *should* do this and do only that; or *should* do that and do, alas, only this. They do not merely recognize their own faults; they inordinately magnify them. Above all, they think a serious failing makes them a total failure. They condemn not only their poor traits, but *themselves,* their entire personhood, for having such unfortunate traits.

One of the worst instances I have ever seen: a woman whose husband kept blatantly regaling her with stories of how many other women he saw and how he had sex with them. When, after driving herself to distraction, she sought the sympathetic ear of one of her male cousins, and started to become attached to him because of his kindness, she began to feel terribly guilty, to look upon herself as the vilest kind of adulteress, and to think that she did not make a fit mother for her children. I had a difficult time showing her that her unrealistic self-demands and her consequent feelings of worthlessness, not her adultery, truly underlay her ceaseless self-criticism.

Guilt and self-blame. People with severe problems usually have severely moralistic codes. They blame others and themselves for innumerable desires and deeds. As Sigmund Freud emphasized, they have particular difficulty accepting their own sex drives. But this often represents only the tip of the iceberg, for they also condemn themselves for many nonsexual deeds. They tend to get too conscientious in their thoughts and too lax in their actions. They know what they *should* do—and don't do it. Then they berate themselves unmercifully.

One of my clients who had the highest standards of

22

personal conduct and honesty obtained a job doing door-to-door selling of encyclopedias. He liked the work because he felt that he could help raise the cultural level of the families to whom he sold, and he began to do very well at the job. After a while, however, he upset himself so much about the possibility of making the slightest exaggerated claim for his product that he spent hours rewording his memorized sales talk. Even that did not satisfy him, and he began to add all kinds of qualifications and hedgings, so that his customers began to feel that he wanted to apologize for even trying to sell them the books. Naturally his sales fell off and, in sheer desperation, he sought psychotherapy. He finally helped himself when he began to see that his phobia against telling any kind of story or half-truth stemmed from his acceptance and perpetuation of his mother's great fear that he would follow in his father's footsteps, cheat at cards, and thereby go "bad."

Supersensitivity and oversuspiciousness. People with disturbances often behave suspiciously. They do not merely believe that others dislike them; they look for, actively ferret out, and seek until they ultimately find this dislike. They feel such underlying guilt about their own behavior that they convince themselves that everyone sees them through their own distorted vision and, consequently, detests them.

A clear example: One of my clients noticed that I sometimes put two fingers over my upper lip and hold them against the under part of my nose. This I do indiscriminately, with clients, friends, intimates. Said this particular woman: "I see that you hold your fingers over your nose. You do this because you think I smell bad, don't you?" "No," I replied, "but obviously *you* think that I (and everyone else) thinks you smell bad." "How did you know?" she asked.

Hostility and resentment. Many "neurotics" behave with hostility and resentment. Hating themselves, they tend to hate others. Feeling that the world unfairly does them in,

23

they think they have to retaliate in kind. Frustrated, largely by their own irrational behavior, they often respond with the common sequel—aggression against the presumably frustrating society and the people in it.

The treasurer of a group to which I once belonged kept getting into difficulties with the other officers of the group because he insisted on doing things in a high-handed, unorthodox manner. When the others complained about his methods he felt most aggrieved, and viewed them as unfair spoilers of his projects. As a result of his frustration—or, actually, of his telling himself that he *must* not get frustrated —he acted with hostility not only toward his fellow officers, but toward almost everyone else. If given the chance, he would complain for hours at a time about politicians, bureaucrats, modern fiction, mothers-in-law, school systems, and a dozen other pet annoyances. He never saw that his hostility did not stem from his disliking interference from others, but from his internally *commanding* that everyone do things his way.

Ingratiation. Many people spinelessly curry favor with others at the expense of their own self-acceptance. In an effort to win love and approval, they slavishly bow to their relatives and associates, abase themselves—and then hate themselves more and feel greater insecurity and rejection. Moreover, because they loathe their own ingratiating tendencies, they frequently try to compensate by reversing themselves and beaming hostility toward those whose favor they seek.

One of my own acquaintances indulges in a typical neurotic pattern in which he apologizes to his wife for everything he does or does not do; then he will verbally slice her to ribbons for some trivial error, such as forgetting to pick up the laundry. Similarly, one of my clients encourages her father to use her as a doormat. Then she complains to me for hours about how nastily he behaves. When I point out

24

to such people that there may exist a connection between how they bow down to others and how they hate these others, they often have trouble seeing how the first of these attitudes can lead to the second. But once they do see the connection, act assertively, and give up their ingratiating behavior, a large part of their hostility vanishes.

Inefficiency and stupidity. "Neurotics," even when they *Inefficiency* achieve at a high level, act inefficiently. Many do things badly or not at all. Others do too much or achieve success the too-hard way—with a needless sacrifice of time, nervous and physical energy, and pleasure. They work unsystematically, without proper planning, or work compulsively, with involved systems that bog them down and promote complications. They block so emotionally that they will not or cannot think their problems through. Or they think them through rationally enough and then continue to act in the same irrational manner as before.

I treated a woman majoring in philosophy and doing exceptionally well. One day she came to me and said that her parents had left their home for a while, and that she kept house so sloppily in their absence that she actually feared an invasion by rats. "Why don't you clean the place?" I asked.

"Oh, but in such lovely weather," she replied, "I'd rather sit in the sun and enjoy myself."

"But you don't weigh up the whole equation," I said. "You don't think logically."

"What do you mean?"

"Well, you measure doing the housework against sitting in the sun and enjoying yourself. Naturally, in terms of that equation, you'll continue to sit in the sun. But the truer equation includes: sitting in the sun—*and* having unpleasant things constantly hang over your head; or doing the housework—*and* feeling free to enjoy yourself later by sitting in the sun, or doing almost anything else you please."

25

"Yes, I guess that sounds about right."

"Now which side adds up to the most enjoyment?"

"I see."

She promptly began cleaning the house.

Self-deceit

Self-deceit and lack of realism. Virtually all "neurotics" lie to themselves and refuse to accept reality. Instead of squarely facing their frustrations, admitting their failings, or unwhiningly accepting the grim facts of life, they tend to rationalize, evade issues, blame others, and construct a picture of the world that contains more poetry than truth.

A physician whom I had known from college days continued to visit me every few years, and each time he arrived he would have in tow a good-looking female companion who obviously had nothing in common with him intellectually. He would take me aside during the course of the evening and long-windedly explain what fine traits she had, her sexual advantages, and how she behaved more desirably than women of his own cultural and intellectual background. I would quietly ask a few pointed questions to indicate my skepticism about his achieving a lasting relationship with her; but he would defend his choice spiritedly. Then, on his next visit, he would tell me how rightly I had guessed about the last woman; but *this* one, now—and he would launch into a highly unrealistic evaluation of his current companion's qualities.

Only after a good many years had passed, and my friend finally had some intensive psychotherapy, did he feel free to admit that his going with the whole series of attractive women resulted from his underlying deep-seated feelings of inadequacy in the presence of those who showed brightness and substance. These inadequacy feelings had led him, via the common route of wishful thinking, into unrealistically assessing his companions and deceiving himself into believing that they had remarkable assets.

Defensıvnss

Defensiveness. Once they begin lying to themselves, "neurotics" set up defense systems against their having to face unpleasant realities. Usually, they devise an elaborate network of devious reactions, and consciously pretend that they feel or act one way when they unconsciously respond to quite a different set of feelings. Some of the common forms of neurotic defensiveness:

Rationalization—Providing a reason for the commission of an act one considers blameworthy. Examples: The mother who has a neurotic urge to criticize her son, but insists that she does so only for his good; the man who collects pornographic literature and insists that he does so only because of his scientific interest in sex.

Compensation—Acting well in one area to set up a smoke screen for neurotically running away from another dangerous area. Examples: The woman who, afraid to go to dances, practically lives in the public library instead, and develops outstanding knowledge of medieval history; the man who develops into a great baseball team manager because he fears he would not excel at playing the game.

Identification—Compensating for one's own weakness by closely allying oneself with someone who appears to have strength. Examples: The coward who believes himself a "real man" because he associates with bullies and bruisers; the somewhat homely teen-age girl who feels at one with a highly attractive female movie star and refuses to acknowledge her own deficiencies.

Projection—Throwing the blame or responsibility for one's own failings onto others. Example: A man who hates his father accuses the father of hating him; or incorrectly views other men as hating their fathers.

Repression—Unconsciously forgetting about aspects of one's own behavior of which one feels ashamed or which one looks upon as painful. Examples: The woman who cannot remember anything about the night she went to bed with a stranger; the fellow who remembers only the tennis games he won and conveniently forgets those he lost.

Resistance—Refusing to face unpleasant facts about oneself, even when they get pointedly brought to one's attention. Examples: The therapy client who refuses to admit that he has hostile feelings toward his mother when his therapist demonstrates that his relations with her have clearly followed a hostile pattern; the card player who insists that he plays well even when he makes many mistakes.

Transference—Unconsciously feeling toward a person attitudes not based on reality, but on that person's having some traits in common with individuals, especially one's parents, to whom one may have previously had attachments. Examples: The teen-ager who, because he resents his parents, may feel rebellious toward teachers, policemen, and other authority figures; the man who loathes his second wife because she has a few traits in common with his mother and his first wife.

Grandiosity—Overcompensating by seeing oneself as having better traits than one actually has because one fears, underneath, that one behaves inadequately. Examples: The revolutionist who, in order to establish himself as kingpin, sets up a group of his own that actually differs little from the group from which he has broken; the man, who, although he lives irresponsibly, thinks that the world owes him a living because of his imagined superiority.

Reaction formation—Refusing to acknowledge feelings (such as anxiety or hostility) that one does not want to face, and unconsciously expressing the reverse emotion. Examples: The mother who really loathes her son, but smothers him with affection and insists she adores him; the fellow who feels insanely jealous of his friend's prowess, but refuses to admit this to himself or to others and, instead, acts as this friend's best press agent.

Refusal to perform—Avoiding or postponing a perform-ance or test one fears failing, and telling oneself one would succeed if one did buckle down to it. Example: The college student who puts off doing his work till the end of the term, takes his exams without having had time to catch up with the work, and then tells himself that if he had worked harder he would have done marvelously.

Rigidity and compulsiveness. "Neurotics" feel unsafe, in-secure. In an effort to attain a greater degree of security, they frequently adopt an arbitrary set of rules and stick to them rigidly. Because they have anxiety about doing the wrong thing, or about letting their thoughts and deeds get beyond their control, they tend to pick certain aspects of life that they *can* easily control and then stick compulsively to these straight and narrow paths. They often devise magical rituals and formulas—such as going through a studied routine before bedtime—to give themselves a feeling that some unknown power protects them as long as they adhere closely to their chosen formulas.

One of the college students I treated took six sharply pointed pencils into every examination and lined them up neatly in front of her. Then she proceeded to ignore them entirely and used a ball-point pen for the exam. She thought that if she temporarily forgot anything she had studied for the exam, the reserve pencils would magically help her recall this reserve material. After she had achieved more confi-dence, as a result of several therapy sessions, she would take her exams without the compulsively arranged extra pencils, for she then felt able to rely on her general ability rather than on a special ritual.

Shyness and withdrawal. Believing that they may easily do the wrong thing and that others will spot their mistakes, numberless "neurotics" act shyly and retreat into various kinds of solitude. Constructively, they may follow solitary occupations such as working alone in a laboratory or in a

29

forest as a ranger. Destructively, they may merely avoid people, stay alone in their rooms, or act as hermits. They thereby draw for themselves one of the frequent neurotic vicious circles: because they fear people they withdraw from society —and thus enhance their fear.

A twenty-two-year-old male had immense difficulty getting up in the morning. When he finally did start for work, he would stand in a corner in the end compartment of the train and face the side of the compartment so that others could not see him. He took his lunch to work and remained alone in his office to eat it. When he returned home at night, he ate quickly and then went right to bed. Initially so shy that he literally would never look other people in the eye, when at last he managed to do this without blushing and quickly averting his gaze, you'd have thought he had just made the varsity football team or won a Phi Beta Kappa key.

Antisocial or psychopathic behavior. Many "neurotics" take a rebellious path from the start, and try to compensate for their underlying feelings of inadequacy by acting as "tough guys" or cynics. A few go to extremes and consistently behave delinquently or criminally. Although some psychologists view these so-called psychopaths as special kinds of warped personalities, my own experience with scores of them convinces me that, at bottom, their "psychopathy" represents a defensive covering used by frequently confused, frightened individuals to harden themselves against underlying feelings of rejection and deep-seated supersensitivity. Relatively few "neurotics" deserve the label "psychopath"; but dig beneath so-called psychopathic behavior and you often find a neurotic (or psychotic) underpinning.

As chief psychologist of the New Jersey Department of Institutions and Agencies, some years ago, I interviewed a young man who had a long series of delinquencies, including burglary, holdups, and stolen cars. At the time I saw him he had just gotten apprehended for shooting his woman friend, crippling her for life, because he jealously objected to her wearing sweaters that revealed her buxom figure to other males. He showed not the slightest remorse about this act, nor about any of the criminal acts he had perpetrated. All told he displayed remarkable coolness.

In the course of the interview I asked this man a few routine questions about his sex history, including any oral genital relations with females. "Whadya mean by asking questions like that?" he bellicosely interrupted. "Whadya think I'd do that for, anyway?"

"You mean," I asked, "that you think such acts wrong?"

"Wrong! I should say so! Besides, whadya think the other guys would say about me if I did things like that? How could I ever face them?"

Behind even the hardest "psychopathic" mien, then, we often find neurotic supersensitivity.

Psychosomatic symptoms and hypochondria. Many physical ailments have a neurotic component. People sometimes worry themselves into sickness by keeping their muscles and nervous systems in a state of hypertension, thus helping to bring on such psychosomatic complaints as ulcers, high blood pressure, asthma, and heart palpitations. Moreover, when they do contract a physical ailment, they sometimes prolong and aggravate it, using it as an excuse for their emotional upsets.

One of my many hypochondriac clients complained that he just could not stop worrying about the possibility of serious illness. If he had a pain in his head, he saw a certain brain tumor. A simple cough convinced him that he had tuberculosis. A stomach twinge set him to thinking of cancer. And whatever he thought he had, he saw as fatal.

"Why do you keep worrying about these illnesses all the time?" I asked.

"Well, because I could die, couldn't I? And at my young age, too, before I've barely lived!"

"Maybe so," I said. "But did it ever occur to you that you spend so much time and energy worrying over the possibility of dying young that you actually give yourself no opportunity to enjoy the one life you'll ever have? Under these conditions, what have you to live for, anyway?"

"Not very much, you make it appear."

"You mean," I said, "*you* make it appear. Only you can wreck your life by worrying over something almost entirely beyond your control."

"I never thought of it that way," said the client. "Maybe you've got something there." And shortly thereafter, he began to think more and worry less.

Crackpotism and bizarreness. Not all "eccentrics," as we previously noted, behave neurotically, but plenty of them do. As they don't tend to get along too well in this world, they frequently try to create a world of their own and acquire all kinds of crackpot, bizarre notions about how to live.

When "neurotics" get sufficiently bizarre and lose sight of reality entirely, we call them "psychotics." We regard neurosis as a reasonably mild evasion of reality; psychosis represents an extreme form of escape from the real world into one of illusion or fantasy. "Psychotics" generally have an even lower estimate of themselves than do "neurotics," and consequently the defenses they erect against fully accepting themselves take on more drama than neurotic defenses, often consisting of hallucinations, extreme projections, godlike feelings, and the like. Or else "psychotics" overaccept their "faults," continually berate themselves, and get into extreme depression.

"Neurotics" may also engage in bizarre behavior, though such behavior does not necessarily suggest the need to get carted off to the nearest mental hospital. The superintendent of the apartment house where I once lived kept inventing schemes for winning at the racetrack. Essentially, his system consisted of doubling his previous bets and keeping on doubling until finally a winner came up. He had considerable intelligence and experience with racing, not to mention the awareness that any such scheme as this might only work when backed by virtually unlimited funds. With limited resources at his disposal, however, he insisted on trying one new scheme after another, and of course he lost heavily. But he so desired to make a killing, to prove his genius to the world and thereby magically erase his tremendous underlying feeling of worthlessness, that he continued to devise bizarre, surefire betting systems.

Depression. A few people manage to compensate well for *Depression* their inner insecurities and remain outwardly content. But average "neurotics" often feel intense depression. They tend to fill themselves with self-pity and pessimism. As Drs. Aaron T. Beck and Paul A. Hauck have shown, depression and neurosis frequently go hand in hand.

A family friend, a sixty-year-old woman, depressed herself as miserably as anyone I have ever seen. Every time she came to visit, her face literally lined with misery, she had copious tears as she described the woeful time she had had during the past few days. Night after night, she reported, she lay awake, sometimes until early morning, crying, sighing, moaning, verbally bewailing her sorrowful lot. The presumed cause of her despair? The fact that her only living son seemed determined to die a bachelor, thus leaving her with no male grandchildren. (Her daughter, mother of two girls, had passed childbearing.) Because this "horrible" situation, she alleged, negated her entire purpose in life, she might just as well never have come into this world. When I attempted to show her that this situation itself could not possibly have caused her depression, but that her unrealistic and childish

33

attitude toward the situation had caused it, she considered me an unfeeling brute who had no understanding of a woman's role in life.

Self-centeredness and inability to love. Most "neurotics" have an inordinate desire to receive, and an infinitesimal willingness to give love. They feel so incessantly concerned with themselves and their own problems that they have neither the time, the energy, nor the inclination truly to care for another person. They often fall violently in love, usually grasping obsessively after individuals whose love they think they need. But they show little ability to care: to want to help others achieve their *own* growth and happiness for their *own* ends.

I particularly remember, in this connection, one of the first girls I dated, as a teen-ager. She, because of what I later began to see as her acute self-downing, had a tremendous "need" for love, adoration, and approval. When she met a boy who she believed would meet her demands, she quickly and violently attached herself to him, and insisted that she loved him passionately. Then, as soon as she discovered that her beloved did not wish to worship her exclusively to bolster her ego, but instead had some deep-seated desires of his own, she took the discovery as an absolute betrayal, insisted that he did not "really" or "truly" love her, and broke up the relationship to seek a new great love. This ceaseless, fruitless search for perfect love has continued, as far as I know, to the present day, through several marriages and innumerable affairs. However, she has never sought, for one, the answer to the question: "Why do I keep demanding amatory perfection?"

Tenseness and inability to relax. Because they preoccupy themselves with constant worry about the rightness or wrongness of their behavior, "neurotics" rarely will relax. As a result, they suffer from a tension which may evidence itself in muscular ailments, poor coordination, or the inability to sit still. Sometimes psychological tension results, and they report that they feel emotionally numb, would like to take out their brains and place them in the refrigerator, or fear something but don't know what. If we did not make a certain amount of effort, we would hardly succeed in doing anything or getting anywhere. But "neurotics" experience unnecessary effort: strain caused by their groundless fears, their overconcerns about what other people think about them.

I saw a young woman who could only with great difficulty describe her tenseness. She felt ashamed that she bit her nails. But aside from this information, she could hardly tell me how she felt. She would vaguely start a sentence: "I don't know what to say—I can't tell you how I feel—I just don't know . . ." Then she would hesitate before taking another stab: "I can't tell—I don't want to do anything. No, I don't mean that: I don't know what I do want to do. I just don't know exactly how to put it . . ."

Only after considerable questioning could I elicit the fact that she felt extremely restless. She thought she could stay in her own room for no more than a few moments; did not feel comfortable even when talking to her parents; would read for only a few pages at a time; did nothing, in fact, for more than a short while without jumping up and wanting to do something else.

Why did this woman feel so tense? Because most of the things she wanted to do, such as championship ice-skating, her parents opposed; and either she refrained from doing them or did them with a feeling of guilt. What she did *not* want to do—including going to art school—her parents virtually insisted upon. So, either she refused to do these things and angered herself about her parents' pressure or she did them and made herself feel guilty. The only independence she let herself achieve she got by actively rebelling against

35

her family. Then she upset herself about her "nasty" rebel-liousness. No wonder she rarely felt relaxed!

Overexcitability and manic tendencies. Some "neurotics" instead of getting depressed make themselves overexcited. Trying to compensate for their (conscious or unconscious) feelings of inadequacy, they act as exhibitionists, overbearing, or life-of-the-party-ish. Others, to avoid facing their own dis-turbances, constantly attempt to keep themselves stimulated by outward forms of excitement; normal conditions of daily life leave them bored and listless.

We find a prime example of neurotic extraversion in the case of a thirty-six-year-old male whose parents largely ignored him as a child to devote most of their attention to his highly talented older sister. Because he still keeps whining about this, he feels he now cannot bear feeling ignored or even unapplauded by anyone. Though not manic, he easily falls into surliness and depression. If he does *not* continually impress people, he thinks they will find him inferior. Enor-mously self-centered, he has little real interest in other people and no main goal aside from showing off. Consequently, he strives incessantly for attention—to find the center of some group. If this group gets into something different and un-conventional—such as playing strip poker—so much the better. He will participate in the attention—and admiration, he believes—that accrue to the group, and he will (literally and figuratively!) outstrip the others. "Anything for excite-ment!" he avers. But he really means: "Anything to divert me from thinking seriously about myself and facing my intense feelings of inferiority!"

Inertia and lack of direction. Many "neurotics" tend to feel unenergetic and to lack definite vital interests. They place themselves on a sort of sitdown strike against life, since they believe that the world owes them a living and should not require them to work hard or to discipline themselves to get the things they want. Deep in their hearts, they do want to strive for something, to realize some goal. But as soon as they meet difficulties in their striving, they give up and withdraw from competition. Then getting back to work comes even harder because it leads to poor accomplishment, which in turn encourages a feeling of hopelessness and more inertia.

One twenty-six-year-old came to see me because of his impotence. We soon discovered that both his father and mother worked exceptionally hard building a large commercial enterprise by devoting almost all their waking hours to it. He resented this, feeling that the time his parents put into the business belonged rightfully to him.

Because of his resentment, he hated work and spent most of his time hanging around poolrooms and bowling alleys. In his sex relations he also refused to "work" at satisfying his partners, and hence made himself impotent. Only after he began facing his sitdown strike against employment and against females did he start working well and displaying sexual adequacy.

Overambitiousness and compulsive striving. Some "neurotics" compensate for their self-flagellation by working themselves practically to death. Not that all hard workers rate as disturbed. In fact, individuals with self-acceptance usually work harder than the average. But "neurotics" overwork because they feel so insecure that they think they *need* fame or fortune; because by constant activity they can distract themselves from some of the psychological pain with which they plague themselves; because work often gives them an excuse to avoid things they terribly fear—for example, engaging in love affairs or attending social gatherings.

A woman of my acquaintance achieved real distinction as a writer of historical novels. She felt depressed, however, and once when I discussed her problems with her she freely

37

admitted that most of her success as a writer had come from very hard work. Where other writers did months of research for a novel, she did years. She spent hour after hour in the library, rewrote her plots and her characterizations again and again, drew involved maps and genealogical tables, and generally so perfected everything she wrote that her readers always marveled at the fineness of her details. And well they might, since these details she wrung, so to speak, from her very life's blood.

She admitted that, although she had had financial and critical success from her teens onward, she had never really done much for herself, for her own happiness. She sought so intently for the highest possible achievement, for getting acclaim, that she rarely took vacations, attended shows and concerts, or relaxed at home. She lived mainly for her work; made herself into a nonentity as a personality.

Escapism and avoidance of responsibility. Instead of facing and working out serious difficulties, "neurotics" frequently see a problem and run. They refuse to discipline themselves or to assume the normal responsibilities of life. Often they attempt to live as perpetual children, and if they marry, they live as child-wives and child-husbands. If they can literally run away from normal exigencies, they do: to a new home, a new job, a new marriage, a new wardrobe. When they cannot actually run, they balk and sulk.

One of my most difficult clients, a young man with a positive genius for avoiding the tasks of life, never kept a job for more than a few weeks and contended that he found the work too hard, the boss impossible, or the hours too long. He never considered marrying any of his many female companions, but saw this one as too demanding, that one as too compliant, and the other as too this or too that. He failed to vote because he considered his city's registration and voting regulations too onerous and time-consuming.

I allowed this client to meander along in therapy for over a year, during which time he gave me countless excuses for his inability to do one thing or another. I kept pointing out that he continually sabotaged himself by his do-nothing attitude. Finally, after I had given him enough rope to hang himself ten times over and he had proceeded to use it for exactly that purpose, he began to stick with one job and to develop a good relationship with one woman. I commended his progress.

"Yes," he said, "I guess I've surprised you. Well, let me tell you the reason for my change. I've worked with you for eighteen months now—which seems rather long for your therapy. But I've learned one thing in those eighteen months, and if I never learn anything else from this process, that one thing will remain with me for the rest of my life."

"What?" I asked.

"Simply that, although I still find getting up and going to work every morning hardly the most pleasurable thing in the world, I now know, and shall remember, that I find *not* working much worse."

"You mean?"

"I mean that while working steadily and assuming certain responsibilities often gives me a pain—though *less* pain as I continue to do so—*not* working and *not* assuming those responsibilities usually brings me far more pain. I waste my time and decrease my present and future enjoyment when I don't work. And I worry so much about what I'd better do that I hardly enjoy the here and now."

Alcoholism and drug addiction. "Neurotics" frequently use alcohol and drugs to escape reality and to temporarily reduce anxiety. Unfortunately, these "escapes" boomerang on their users, since they help create increased disturbance and hence lead to a desire for still larger doses.

Even when drugs and alcohol temporarily work, the

39

users know that, without their aid, they cannot do the things they fear, so they obtain no increased confidence. Indeed, they usually hate themselves all the more for using these self-defeating "tranquilizers," and the usual vicious neurotic circle results.

A man with typical alcoholic symptoms had an excellent position but also had a somewhat rigid supervisor. He liked the work but hated the supervisor. He reluctantly faced this hatred, however, because it too closely resembled his feelings toward his own father, a person with traits similar to his supervisor's. To avoid this conflict, he frequently would not show up for work, giving himself the excuse that he did not feel well.

His absences got so frequent that he made himself feel ashamed of phoning in his excuses. Whereupon his supervisor would call to find out why he had not shown up. Afraid to face these calls, he would drink himself into insensibility so that he could not hear the phone, or would sit staring at it while he counted the number of rings. Then, when it finally stopped ringing, he would feel so ashamed that he would go on a binge for several days. After he sobered up, he would go back to work for a while, but then begin the same pattern of absenteeism and drinking. When he faced his unconscious hostility toward his father and realized he had transferred these resentments to his boss, he saw what he typically did' to anger himself and to express his anger. With the aid of rational-emotive therapy, he then attacked his own childish beliefs—especially the belief that he *should* have a loving, kind father-boss. And when at last he stopped condemning himself and others, and instead only criticized and tried to change his and their behavior, he lost his compulsion to drink.

Self-downing and self-punishment. In addition to downing themselves for their poor traits, some "neurotics" damn and punish themselves for their main "sin"—their neurosis. Starting with unrealistic, perfectionist assumptions that create feelings of general inadequacy, they actualize their self-fulfilling prophecies and do things they think they "cannot help" doing. Then, noting their "inevitable" weakness or "badness," they do something weaker or meaner. This leads them to flagellate *themselves* more, instead of only judging their poor *behavior*.

As a grim example of self-whipping, I remember an administrative assistant at an institution where I worked. He felt marital sex relations permissible only when they resulted in childbearing. Always on the brink of financial insolvency, however, he and his wife could not afford to add to their brood of four children, and therefore they regularly employed birth-control procedures. The husband felt so guilty about this that he would frequently quarrel with his wife during the day, thus making it almost impossible for them to have satisfactory sex relations at night. On the few occasions when he succeeded in having intercourse, he managed either to perform ineffectually or unenjoyably.

One of my clients who frantically tried to lose weight kept backsliding on her diet. Often, after overeating a little, she deliberately punished herself by going on to eat half a box of candy or drink several bottles of beer. When she took a more realistic attitude toward human failings and accepted *herself* with her foolish behavior, she made real headway with dieting.

The main message of this chapter boils down to this: "Neurotics" theoretically have the capacity to act effectively, creatively, and free from sustained anxiety and hostility. However, because they hold irrational, unrealistic assumptions—such as the philosophy that they *must* win universal approval, that they *should not* get frustrated, or that they've committed a horror if they fail at something important—they create and sustain (mainly by constant negative self-talk) disturbed and self-harming emotions.

When "neurotics" manufacture overconcern, rage, guilt,

41

feelings of worthlessness, and depression, they can choose to consciously experience these self-sabotaging emotions or set up unconscious defenses against them. Their defenses may include self-deceit, projection, rationalization, evasiveness, psychosomatic complaints, alcoholism, drug addiction, anti-social behavior, compensation, or other forms of escapism.

Often, because they have general philosophies of damnation and atonement, "neurotics" first hate themselves for not displaying the perfection they think they should display. Then, once they develop disturbed feelings or ineffectual behavior, they additionally loathe themselves for their neuroses. A vicious circle thereby arises: as a result of unrealistic beliefs they behave badly, condemn themselves further for thus behaving, and consequently add greatly to their emotional woes!

3

How Emotional Disturbances Originate

To live successfully with emotional disturbance, you'd better know something about its origins. Let us now look into its whys and hows.

No one, as far as we know, gets born neurotic, although some inherited factors may make it easier for one person to grow up disturbed, while another person, living under more harrowing conditions, develops healthily.

We learn neurotic behavior as a result of three main influences: (1) our inborn tendencies to think, feel, and act; (2) the environmental and cultural circumstances in which we get reared; and (3) the ways we choose to act—or *condition ourselves* to the things we experience.

Neurosis, like syphilis and the measles, rates as a kind of social ailment. We partly catch it from our parents and from those around us. We get raised by other humans and they help teach us neurotic behavior. But we also decide to accept—or, occasionally, reject—these nutty teachings.

We first propel ourselves toward neurosis with the attitudes toward ourselves and others that we pick up (or *make* up) in childhood. We acquire irrational attitudes, believe that certain conditions (such as receiving love or doing well) *should* or *must* exist, and that certain other conditions (such as getting frustrated or forced to shift for oneself) *should not* or *must not* exist. As a result of our unrealistic ideas, we usually wind up by hating ourselves and others.

Your ideas about yourself and others you partly acquire or learn, originally, from your parents or other people who wield influence in your early life. Much of what we call your *self* comes not just from *you;* it derives in part from your interaction with other humans: your *social* self. You learn that you have certain qualities that distinguish you from others, and you learn this *from* these others. Thus, you learn to identify one type of man as "handsome" and another as "ugly"; one kind of woman as "bright" and another "stupid." And you learn that on various scales of handsomeness-ugliness or brightness-stupidity you yourself stand at a certain point, while others stand at different points.

This learning, incidentally, appears somewhat relative or accidental, since you may learn something different if you happen to get raised in one part of the world, or in one family, rather than in another. In one community, for example, you may learn to regard dark skins as "handsome" and that you, having a very dark skin, qualify as very "handsome." But if you get raised in another community, you may see people with dark skins as "ugly" and yourself, having a very dark skin, as very "ugly."

Therefore, your attitude toward yourself, your self-concept, tends to depend upon the concepts prevalent in the particular community, region, and family in which you grow up. If you come to value intelligence and beauty as worthwhile traits, then find that you have them, you will tend to look upon yourself as "good" and to have a favorable self-concept. But if you get raised to believe yourself stupid and ugly, you will tend to look upon yourself as "bad" and to have a poor self-concept. Whether you actually have intelligence or good looks may have little to do with how you judge your-

self, for you may unthinkingly accept others' views, even
though they happen to have little or no truth.

Your early self-concepts, in other words, usually depend
on the attitudes that others take toward you or the propa-
ganda with which they surround you. If those important to
you generally blame you, you will probably blame yourself. If
they consistently accept you, you will tend to accept yourself.
This does not mean that your early self-concept remains absolutely final and crucial. You can, later in life, change it for better or worse. But this early self-concept has considerable importance, and you do tend to make it the pattern for later
attitudes and behavior.

Because in our society we have considerably more *don't's*
than *do's* for children, and because we consistently tell them
that they have behaved wickedly or naughtily when they
dirty our rugs, kick over our vases, or refuse to go to sleep on
time, we tend to encourage millions of our youngsters—in
fact, virtually all of them—to have fairly negative concepts of
their behavior. Then, because humans tend to confuse their
traits with *themselves* and to falsely conclude "If my *trait*
stinks, *I* am a stinker," many children wind up with poor
self-concepts. These negative concepts, or feelings of inadequacy and worthlessness, form one of the central cores of
later neuroses.

Putting it differently, we might say that we mainly tend
to control children's behavior today, not by beating or punishing them, but by explaining to them that certain of their acts
prove "naughty" or "bad" and that no one, especially their
parents, will love or approve of *them* if they continue to
do these *things*. Because children (and adults!) easily overgeneralize, we thereby help them to accept several false propositions: (a) that they must act well and thereby earn their
"goodness"; (b) that they should consider it disastrous if they
behave badly; (c) that they have to win the love and ap-

proval of virtually everyone; and (d) that they should feel awful if they don't.

If children devoutly accept these premises and grow up without modifying them, they virtually doom themselves to neurosis. They will spend the rest of their days trying to do the impossible: always trying to appear "good people" and invariably win the love and approval of everyone. And, since they will not succeed at these impossible tasks, and will tend to fear they will later fail even when they *now* succeed, they will acquire deep-seated feelings of inadequacy and self-hatred, and often low frustration tolerance and hostility, too.

Most of the people who come to see me about their difficulties have above-average intelligence and ability, since therapy still largely appeals to individuals with higher educational backgrounds. Yet almost all my clients convince themselves that they have serious unchangeable deficiencies.

A college student, unusually tall, handsome, and intelligent, composed music and painted so well that his teachers predicted he would develop into an outstanding craftsman in both fields. Yet he not only considered himself so unworthy of female companionship that he never tried to date women, but he also carried on homosexual activities with the most stupid and least cultured "rough trade" he could find, for fear that other companions would not accept him.

This student had a social-register mother who turned over his upbringing almost entirely to nursemaids and servants and who never stopped criticizing her son whenever the boy did anything "improper" or "unmanly." On one occasion, when he imbibed too much at one of her parties and fell asleep on a bench in the patio and wet his pants, she unceremoniously woke and roundly scolded him in front of the guests. Another time, she found him playing in her clothes closet, and falsely accused him of spying on her undressing.

To make matters worse, this student's father, rarely at

46

home, kept having obvious affairs with other women. He finally divorced his wife when the son was nine and showed no interest in seeing him again, even ignoring invitations to his grade school and prep school graduations. The main picture that the son took of himself agreed with his parents' views. He saw himself as a troublesome individual who merited no particular love or attention.

This young man objectively acknowledged that he did well at this thing or that, including his composing and painting; but he still saw himself as a worthless, essentially unlovable person. It surprised him that I, as his therapist, found him acceptable, apart from his accomplishments; and, partly through this unconditional acceptance, he began to stop his self-hating. Mainly, however, I actively taught him that he did have a self-chosen right to life and enjoyment no matter how often he failed or who thought ill of him.

If you reach maturity with severe feelings of self-blame, you can do several constructive things. You can, for example, examine the origins of your negative self-concepts and realize that you partly picked them up from the erroneous teachings of your early teachers and partly from your own tendency to incorrectly identify your *acts* as *you*. Then you can set about de-propagandizing yourself by consistently refusing to label yourself as "bad," even though you perform some heinous deeds. Since, like all humans, you have great fallibility, you may question the assumption that you should behave perfectly and infallibly. Finally, though you'd better admit you do certain "bad" or self-defeating things, you can ask yourself "Must I *always* do 'good' ones?" and "Do I *have* to win others' approval for doing well?"

Even with these constructive approaches to dealing with the problem of believing in your wickedness or worthlessness, you may find it hard to take these steps. For you, as a human, tend to believe not merely in the importance, but in the absolute sacredness—the *all*-importance—of good deeds and of others' approval. And you tend to feel so panicked when in danger of committing "bad" deeds or of meriting disapproval that you often freeze and almost lose the ability to do anything constructive. Instead, you often take the "neurotic" path and strive desperately to keep winning others' favor, even at the expense of refusing to do what you really want to do in the one life you'll ever have.

One of my clients, the only son of parents who firmly adhered to a group with extremist views, cared nothing for the tenets of this group. But he cared very much for the approval of his parents, who insisted that he participate as an active member of it. Whenever he thought of changing to another group, he made himself terribly anxious about losing the love of his parents, and as a result he invariably returned to the fold—and loathed himself for giving up his independent beliefs.

When confronted by his friends with the fact that he did not really believe in his parents' ideals, this client would insist that he did believe in them, and would cite his past services to their group. But, somehow, when it came to attending political rallies, he usually felt ill just before the meeting, or fell asleep in the midst of it, or otherwise managed not to participate actively. Still, every time he attempted to quit the group, doubts about his decision overwhelmed him and, until his therapy sessions had gotten well under way, he remained in the fold. When he finally decided that doing what he truly enjoyed had more importance to him than having his parents' approval, his anxiety disappeared.

Many—perhaps most—people refuse to squarely face the issue of self-downing. They erroneously believe that by winning the nod of others, they can overcome the feelings of inadequacy with which they indoctrinated themselves. This belief seems foolhardy for several reasons. First of all, feelings of inadequacy actually *stem from* people's dire needs for approval; and so the more they think they have to have other people's love or affection, the greater the feelings of worthlessness they feel. At bottom, people berate themselves because they *think* they must have others accept them, and they fear they will not earn this acceptance. Consequently, the more they need it, the more inferior they feel about its absence.

Secondly, attempting to bolster your self-esteem by winning the love of others utilizes a hazardous means toward a questionable end. If nine people accept you fully, and you begin to feel confident because of their acceptance, you can never count on how the tenth person will react. And, even if you do win everyone's love, you can never know how long you will retain it. Self-acceptance, therefore, that depends largely on what *others* think, rather than on your own decision to discover what *you* enjoy and to enjoy it, builds "esteem" on shifting sands.

A young woman, after seeing me for a few sessions, came one day pleading pathetically, "Please, Dr. Ellis, tell me what to do. I keep meeting new people all the time, and whenever I meet them I immediately try to impress them with my goodness. Naturally, after I act like this for a few minutes, and practically stand on my head to show people how brightly and charmingly I behave, they probably say to themselves, 'Boy, how idiotic! Who does she think she can fool?' And then I notice their reactions and I make an even greater effort to impress them. I always wind up by making a complete fool of myself. I know exactly how I do it while I keep at it, but I just can't stop myself. What can I do?"

"Do you realize," I asked, "what you want me to do?"

"No. What?"

"You really want me to arrange things somehow so that everyone you meet immediately loves you."

"Yes, I guess so. I really do."

"But what you ask me to do won't work, of course—for at least two important reasons. In the first place I can hardly induce anyone—let alone everyone—to love and approve of you."

"No, I guess you can't."

"Moreover, suppose I *could* help you gain the love of everyone you met. Suppose I had a magic wand, and just by waving this wand I could arrange things so that whenever you meet a new person, this individual will immediately love you and know you as a fine person. Why, I would have done you the greatest disservice that one human can do for another! I'd have helped you feel disturbed for the rest of your life."

"What do you mean?"

"Exactly what I said. The very core of your emotional disturbance, like the core of virtually anyone's, consists of your dire *need* for love, your irrational belief that you simply *must* get love and from almost everyone you meet. This constitutes one of the main cores of neurosis. And as long as you think that way, you will feel upset. If I catered to this sickness of yours—if I gave you what you mistakenly think you must have—your disturbance would continue indefinitely."

"You mean that if I want to gain emotional health, I'd better rid myself of the need for approval by everyone I meet? Without surrendering this 'need,' I won't improve?"

"Right! Psychotherapy doesn't help you, as so many people assume, to win everyone's love and approval. It helps you, instead, to get along well in this world *whether or not* other people adore you. Once you accept the fact that you can enjoy yourself even in relatively hostile surroundings, then you won't let anything bother you too much. As long as you believe that happiness depends on what *other* people think, you will tend to doom yourself to misery and depression. Neurosis largely consists of the foolish belief that the world will come to an end unless certain people love you immediately and forever."

"I see," said my client. And, eventually, she really did see, and made a remarkable improvement in her behavior and her feeling.

Most people, however, do not see that winning the love of others has less value than choosing to seek their own enjoyment. They go through their entire lives missing one of the most significant lessons a human can learn—namely, that you generally achieve happiness not by gaining the approval of others, but by mastering, by your own effort and self-discipline, difficult tasks or problems. People usually enjoy creativity. Unless you get vitally absorbed in something—art, science, agriculture, raising a family, playing a good ball game, or what you will—you probably will not have too much fulfillment. Happiness largely stems from creative activity: from intense absorption in some persons or things, rather than from others' involvement in you.

"Neurotics," alas, almost invariably find themselves in a vicious circle creatively. Feeling inferior, and believing they desperately need the approval of others, they fear trying creative activity because they feel they may fail and thereby reap disapproval. Because they fear trying, they don't practice doing things; and lacking practice, they lose out on skills. They then doubly convince themselves that they lack worth and that they cannot do anything well. This leads to further inaction, failure, and self-depreciation.

Negative feedback also results from "neurotics'" attitudes toward their imperfections. Feeling that they cannot do certain things, they have a low level of aspiration. But a direct relationship exists between level of aspiration and performance. If you believe that you can easily broad-jump nine feet, you usually approach or achieve this mark. But if you er-

51

roneously believe that you can jump only eight feet, you will achieve no more than that.

"Neurotics," believing that they will do poorly in this or that task, almost invariably do as poorly as they believe they will. Then they turn right around and say: "See? That proves that I can't do it." Actually, it proves nothing of the sort, but that they have no confidence and that achievement often depends on confidence.

Anxiety, moreover, usually sabotages efficiency. If you have great fear about speaking well, or reading quickly, or playing the piano, you will devote only a small part of your energy and concentration trying to master such a field. Instead, you will spend time asking: "How should I rate myself? Does my audience accept my performance?" And in so concentrating on *how* rather than on *what* you do, you will tend to do poorly.

By the same token, if you feel others oppose you, you may act in an unfriendly, hostile manner to these others. Then, of course, they may quite understandably turn against you and you take this as further "proof" of your original hypothesis!

"Neurotics" get themselves into another kind of vicious circle by feeling inadequate, erecting some defense—such as withdrawing, rebelling, or rationalizing—against their feelings of inadequacy, and then hating themselves for using this defense. Although a few neurotic defenses, such as compensation, lead to socially approved behavior, most lead to social disapproval. And individuals, who felt so inadequate in the first place that they drove themselves to use such defenses, now feel even more ineffectual *because* they use them. Thus, a great many of my clients severely condemn themselves for having neuroses—when their neuroses resulted from their habitual attitude of self-condemnation.

A common tragedy exists on what we call the secondary level of neurosis, that often represents an even greater tragedy than the primary neurosis. Consider an example. Norbert felt weak and ugly, that males did not like him because of his physical weakness, and that women got repulsed by his homeliness. Actually, he had relatively little of the puniness or ungainliness he *thought* he had; and he flagellated himself about his "failings."

Because of his poor estimate of himself, Norbert avoided games and exercises, especially those that might reveal to others his undeveloped body and lack of prowess. He also neglected his appearance, feeling that he could do nothing to improve it. He made it obvious that he did not care about good looks.

As a result of avoiding physical exercise and neglecting his appearance, Norbert actually got inept at sports and looked weak. Some of the fellows, consequently, commented about his lack of physical prowess and these comments eventually got back to him—encouraging him to believe all the more in his hopeless weaknesses.

To defend himself against the unkind observations of others, Norbert began to avoid polite society and to hang around with a group of "neurotics," who did considerable drinking and gambling and kept having minor run-ins with the police. Defensively, he soon began to think this behavior "great stuff." But he also realized that many people disapproved of drinking and that he could not gain general acceptance by these means. On the contrary, most people liked him even less.

Finally, Norbert began to down himself more for his neurotic behavior—his drinking and gambling—than he originally had for his weakness and his poor looks. He felt more inadequate than ever. When he finally saw me, he had gotten involved with a dope-peddling ring, and only a strong psychological recommendation saved him from serving a term in prison.

Soon after I saw Norbert at the New Jersey State Diagnostic Center, I had therapy sessions in New York with Jane, who had just left a girls' reformatory where she had gotten confined for sexual promiscuity leading to an illegitimate pregnancy and a self-induced abortion. At the time I saw her, Jane had just turned sixteen.

Jane originally disturbed herself after her parents, themselves serious "neurotics," neglected her badly and went off for long vacations together while leaving her in the charge of an unsympathetic relative. After several years of this sort of treatment, she whined frequently and acted destructively. Among other things, she did badly in school, although she had always shown superior intelligence in diagnostic tests.

At the reformatory Jane continued to do poorly in school and therefore received training in menial work, which she loathed. She knew that she wanted some higher level activity —such as TV script-writing—but because of her school failures, she rated herself totally stupid and incapable of doing anything except the very work she hated. She then felt more inadequate and disturbed.

Here we have a girl who originally failed academically because of her severe emotional problems. Then she took her academic failure as proof of her own stupidity. Then she got still more disturbed from seeing this "proof." When I first talked to Jane, I found that the original cause of her neurosis —her supersensitivity to her father's and mother's rejection— no longer particularly bothered her, since by this time she had inured herself to their rejection, and even had some insight into their disturbances. But her *secondary* neurosis—her feelings of inadequacy about her original neurotic symptoms (failing at school)—remained with her and continued to plague her until she received therapy.

So it often happens: people surmount the first "cause" of their neurotic symptoms and learn to accept the original circumstances, such as parental rejection, which led them to create these symptoms. But the symptoms themselves get viewed as disapproved behavior, for which they condemn themselves. This condemnation produces woeful feelings of inadequacy, which in turn encourage new neurotic symptoms.

Another example: One of my clients hated himself so much because of his reactions to the continual nagging of his mother, that he stuttered fearfully during the day and lay awake at night worrying about his day's behavior. After a while, even though his mother accepted him and stopped her nagging, he remained anxious about his stuttering and insomnia.

He finally felt so disturbed about his neurotic symptoms that his sense of inadequacy increased, and he stuttered more and slept less. His primary neurosis thus provided a focal point for the starting of a secondary neurosis; and his secondary disturbance brought more misery than the primary one ever had. Until he came for therapy, he made his neurotic circle more vicious and wider, enveloping more and more of his personality in its destructive sweep.

Does neurosis arise solely from feelings of inadequacy and self-hatred? Not exactly. It may result from one or more major irrational ideas, several of which lead not only to feelings of worthlessness or lack of self-confidence, but also to exaggerated feelings of anxiety, hostility, and low frustration tolerance—which we can also include under the heading of neurosis.

What major irrational assumptions or philosophies lead people into neurotic behavior? In studies of my clients (see the Bibliography at the end of this book) I have found that the main irrational ideas you may believe include:

You *must* have approval or love from almost everyone for almost everything you do.

You *have* to display considerable competence, adequacy,

and success in important respects, else your worth or value diminishes.

You *should* condemn yourself severely for your serious mistakes and wrongdoings.

You *should* damn others for their bad behavior, and get upset about their errors and stupidities.

Because a certain thing once strongly affected your life, it *should* indefinitely affect it; because your parents or society taught the acceptance of certain traditions, they *must* now strongly influence you.

If you would like to get the things you value, you *should* get them, and if you can't, you have fallen victim to catastrophe. You *shouldn't* have to put off present pleasures for future gains.

You can more easily avoid than face life's difficulties and responsibilities and still not seriously defeat yourself.

External events cause your emotional reactions and you therefore have virtually no control over these emotions.

You *must* ceaselessly worry over potentially dangerous or injurious things, and your anxiety will then prevent their occurrence.

We may summarize these notions by saying that when you believe that the things you *prefer* or *would like* to happen *should* or *must* occur, and that you have to find life *horrible* or *awful* when they do not, you think, emote, and act irrationally. Why? Because you often cannot change unpleasant and unwanted reality. Because if you sanely view an obnoxious situation, you will try to change it or, if it seems unchangeable, accept it. Making yourself thoroughly upset about an annoying condition will not only fail to improve the condition but usually helps make it considerably worse.

Note that you (and others) tend to hold unrealistic, irrational ideas that create neurosis unconsciously rather than consciously. You often consciously know it makes no sense

56

for you to expect almost everyone to love you, to expect to do things well all the time, to refuse to stand any frustration, or to seriously worry about all threatening possibilities. But, underneath, you firmly and deeply believe this nonsense. Unconsciously, you keep telling yourself that you *should* have love, *must* do well, *ought not* to get frustrated, *should* panic over possible accidents, and the like. Your conscious views, therefore, may seriously conflict with your unconscious values and philosophies. Since you construct the latter unrealistically, you sooner or later feel upset and begin to act neurotically.

To make the workings of emotional disturbance crystal-clear, I frequently outline them in terms of the A-B-Cs of rational-emotive therapy. At point C (an emotional *consequence*), your close female friend, let us say, feels exceptionally hurt and depressed and continues to feel this way for a long period of time—perhaps practically all her life. Her feelings of hurt and depression keep occurring and remaining, she says, because at point A (a series of *activating events* or *activating experiences*) she frequently tries to establish a permanent relationship with a man she likes and he completely rejects her.

Since as soon as she gets rejected at point A, she immediately feels profoundly depressed at point C, she humanly —but wrongly!—concludes that A causes C. She tells you, in fact, "Tom rejected me and that hurt me very much. It depressed me severely to get rejected again like that."

If you have some knowledge of rational-emotive therapy (RET), you immediately know that she has made a wrong conclusion. For A virtually never causes C: since Tom's rejecting her, an external event, could hardly get into her gut and *cause* it to throb with hurt and depression. It might *contribute* to such cause; but could hardly *make* her feel depressed.

What, then, *does* cause C? Obviously—if you think about it—B. B represents your friend's *belief system about* A. And, if you know your RET well, you realize that she most probably has two important beliefs about A: a rational (or sensible) and an irrational (or foolish) belief.

Her rational belief (rB) says: "How unfortunate that Tom rejected me! I wish he hadn't. His rejection frustrates me considerably—gives me what I don't want—and I'd better do something, if I can, to overcome it: to win him back or to find someone else (such as Dick or Harry!) who will accept me and give me what I want." If she stayed with this rational belief, and really believed nothing more than this, she would tend to feel quite sorry, annoyed, sad, irritated, and frustrated —but hardly hurt and depressed.

What, then, really causes her depression? Answer, in RET terms: her irrational beliefs (iBs) about the activating experience (A) in her life. To wit: (1) "I find it *awful* that Tom has rejected me!" (2) "I *can't stand* this kind of love rejection!" (3) "I *should* have acted so beautifully with him that he could *never* reject me." (4) "And since I didn't do what I *should* have done, I exist as a slob, an incompetent, a pretty *rotten person.*"

What makes this second set of beliefs irrational or foolish? Their *shoulds* or *musts.* The magical *demands* your friend makes of herself and the universe. Her refusal to accept grim reality; and her whining and whining about its unpleasant aspects.

For if you go to point D—*disputing* of irrational beliefs— you could ask your hurt and upset friend:

(1) "What makes it *awful* that Tom rejected you?" Answer: Nothing makes it awful! Getting rejected certainly brings about disadvantage, inconvenience, and frustration. But to call something *awful* (or *terrible* or *horrible*) really means that it has *more than* disadvantage or unpleasantness

about it; and that because it proves so frustrating, it *should* not, *must* not exist. But, of course, it *does* exist; and your friend had better accept its unpleasant existence and stop *defining* it as *awful*.

(2) "Where can you produce evidence that you *can't stand* getting rejected?" Answer: Your friend can't produce such evidence. She may never *like* or *enjoy* rejection; but it will hardly *kill* her. She can, in fact, stand virtually anything that occurs in her life, until the time she keels over and dies. If she insists that she doesn't *like* rejection, or even *enormously* dislikes it, she remains sensible. But as soon as she declares that she *can't stand* what she dislikes, she believes utter drivel, and almost inevitably upsets herself by believing it.

(3) "Prove that you *should* have done what you didn't do with your friend, in order to get accepted by him." Answer: Again, she can't! For when she says "I *should* have done anything," she means (i) "It would have proved better had I done it" and (ii) "Therefore, a law of the universe exists that says that I *must* do what would have proved better." Although the first of these statements seems correct, can the second one ever get solidly established? Hardly!

(4) "How does it follow that since you didn't do what you supposedly *should* have done, you now exist as a slob, an incompetent, a pretty *rotten person?*" Answer: It doesn't! First of all, as we have just seen, she can't prove that she *should* have acted better with her male friend; so any deduction she makes from this unprovable statement can only turn out to be, at best, an illogical deduction from an unprovable, and most probably invalid, premise. Secondly, for her to exist as a slob, an incompetent, a rotten person, she would have to (i) act rottenly in the past, present, and future; (ii) *inevitably* act rottenly; and (iii) get utterly damned, by some deity or essence of the universe, for acting rottenly. None

of these three propositions seems verifiable. Consequently, the entire concept of her existing as a slob, an incompetent, or a rotten person appears to be a ridiculous overgeneralization, which has little or no possibility of getting proven.

By helping your friend, then, clearly see the A-B-Cs of her feelings of hurt and depression—how *she* creates these feelings herself and how they do not merely *occur* in her gut after some obnoxious experience or event appears in her life at point A—you can show her how to understand herself, to assume responsibility for her feelings, and to refuse to cop out by blaming external people and events for her emotional overreactions. Then, by helping her go on to D—disputing of her own irrational beliefs (iBs)—you can frequently aid her to acquire a new *effect* (E).

The first effect (E) she would acquire would consist of a new philosophic or *cognitive* effect (cE): namely, the revised idea that "I will keep finding it quite unfortunate when a person I care for rejects me for some of my inadequacies and will not relate to me on the level that I would like to relate. But that unfortunateness won't kill me; in fact, I can still live happily, and enjoy myself in other ways, without his accepting me. Tough!—but not *awful*. No matter how many times I get rejected by those I care for, I still want what I want—acceptance—and I think I'll keep trying to get it until I most probably do. And if I never do, that will prove really tough. But never horrible or terrible! And my failing will never make me into a rotten person!"

When she comes to this kind of cognitive effect (cE), your friend will also tend to have a pronounced *behavioral* effect (bE): namely, the *feelings* of sorrow, regret, and frustration rather than those of hurt, depression, and despair; and the *actions* of looking determinedly for someone else with whom she can enjoyably relate.

By using the A-B-Cs of rational-emotive therapy in this

manner, you yourself can understand almost anyone's serious emotional problems; and frequently you can help people understand themselves and do something about disputing their irrational beliefs and changing them—and the self-defeating emotions and behaviors to which they usually lead. You can also, of course, apply these A-B-Cs, and the disputing at D that can follow them, to your own emotional upsets, and can frequently directly deal with them, stop them before they go too far, and improve or eliminate them after you have let them get under way for a period of time.

Do any serious emotional problems exist that you cannot place in the A-B-C framework? Possibly, but it remains questionable whether they truly can get labeled "emotional." Dyslexia, for example, afflicts a good many individuals, especially children. It constitutes a form of disturbance that prevents them from reading too well, and may encourage them to turn into absolute nonreaders. Largely, however, we find it a neurological rather than an emotional disorder: for some people seem born with a peculiar kind of nervous system that predisposes them to have dyslexia. Once people get afflicted with this disorder, they *then* can easily upset themselves about it—by telling themselves (at point B, their belief system) that it feels *awful* to remain a poor reader; that they can't stand it; that they *shouldn't* have that affliction; and that they exist as incompetents, or rotten people, for having it.

At this point these people have both a neurological *and* an emotional problem. And, as you can easily see, their emotional problem follows the A-B-C pattern of human disturbance, even though their original neurological difficulty may have had nothing to do with their *awfulizing*. So not all "personality" difficulties fit into the A-B-C framework. Some of them really prove more physical or neurological than emotional. But what we normally label an emotional upset—or a neurosis—does stem from people's belief systems—from their

61

awfulizing and catastrophizing about the obnoxious activating experiences (A's) that occur in their lives. And such emotional problems can get understood and eliminated by effective use of the A-B-Cs of RET.

What about deep-lying complexes such as the Oedipus complex? How do they fit into the neurotic picture?

These unconscious complexes do not cause neurosis, but represent (or result from) serious conflicts in values and ideas. Take the Oedipus complex, for example. According to Freud and his followers, this arises because a young boy lusts after his mother, wants to have sex with her, fears his father will punish him for his desires, and therefore panics and feels hostile to his father (and other authority figures) and guilty in relation to his mother (and other maternal images).

Suppose that we examine a particular individual and discover that he actually has an Oedipus complex and that he therefore behaves neurotically. The question remains: *Why* does he have such a complex? Did his birth (as Freud thought) virtually doom him to acquire it? No! His complex stems from rather than causes his neurotic pattern. If, for instance, he lusted after his mother and believed lust *natural* and *good* instead of *unnatural* and *bad,* would he truly have a complex about it? Or if he believed lust bad but never viewed himself as a "bad person" for having it, would he then develop any upsetting complex? Of course not!

His Oedipus complex, therefore, does not stem from the *fact* that he lusts after his mother, but from his *beliefs,* his *attitudes,* about these facts. Even if his parents and his culture solidly indoctrinate him with such Oedipal beliefs, he hardly has to accept and perpetuate them! Voilà—he has a complex only if he *chooses* to have one!

Neurosis, then, does not arise from the unfortunate happenings, dangers, or frustrations that often beset our lives, but from our own irrational, unrealistic ideas or views about things and the way they supposedly *should* or *must* turn out. Once we have perfectionist ideologies, one or two major results (as noted in the previous chapter) almost inevitably occur. Either we make ourselves unnecessarily miserable (for example, depressed, guilty, or anxious) and/or we set up defenses against consciously experiencing emotional pain (for example, we rationalize, project, lie, take to alcohol or drugs, or compensate). In other words, neurosis includes: (1) feelings of needless misery or (2) overinhibited, compulsive, or overimpulsive behavior, often designed to cover up such misery. Its main causes? Irrational ideas!

When people experience extraordinary, intense, or prolonged despair, anxiety, or hostility, or when they have unusually rigid defenses and resort to hallucinations, paranoid thinking, extreme inertia, or other unusual escapes from reality, they may get labeled "psychotic" rather than "neurotic." "Psychotics" have such severe emotional problems that they almost always can use intensive professional treatment.

But the majority of people with emotional difficulties usually get the "neurotic" label. If these "neurotics" have understanding and help, they can improve considerably in most instances.

4

Some Basic Factors in Emotional Upsets

Must humans acquire deep-seated feelings of inade-quacy or low frustration-tolerance early in their lives so that they then have a predisposition toward neurosis? Theoreti-cally, no. We can presumably raise children so that they fully accept themselves, do not get obsessed about winning others' approval, and accept life's difficulties without whining or retreating.

In practice, however, many forces encourage the de-velopment of severe inadequacy feelings and emotional up-set. Among them these:

Parental models. If your parents act inadequately and spinelessly, you may tend to identify with them and imitate them in important ways. Thus, you may feel ashamed of them, may believe you come from inferior stock, and define yourself as "bad."

Mothers (and sometimes fathers) frequently ask me: "What can I do, Dr. Ellis, to help my child? I would do any-thing if you would only tell me exactly what."

To the mother of a fourteen-year-old girl who asked this

question, I replied: "You say you really want to help your daughter stop fearing people and teach her how to make friends. Fine. But did you ever stop to think how you and your husband behave in this regard? From what you've told me, you fear joining your local church group because you think you don't quite measure up to the other people in the group. And your husband, you say, even though he hates it, has stayed at the same job for years, largely because he terrifies himself about getting interviewed for a new one. No wonder your daughter fears people, when her own parents show her, by deed as well as attitude, that they think contact with others frightening!"

"You think we should do something about ourselves, then?"

"Not should, but had better. You can probably best help your daughter by helping yourselves. If you cultivate your *own* garden more adequately, she may see by your good example that she can cultivate hers. But as long as *you* set her a poor example, how can you expect her to do better?"

Parental models can have exceptional importance in the life of a child. Parents who act ineffectually and inadequately can help their children feel severe self-deprecation. And those who catastrophize about frustrations may raise "spoiled brats" who, well on into adulthood, behave similarly.

Early rejection. You can encourage children to feel inferior by rejecting them: by showing that you hate them (rather than their behavior). For if the members of their own family devalue youngsters, how can they readily value their own aliveness and cultivate joy?

I knew a couple who had a fairly attractive child whom most relatives and friends of the family liked on sight, made a great fuss over, and significantly favored. The couple also had a rather unattractive younger child, who received relatively little attention.

The younger child actually had greater intelligence and ability to do schoolwork than the older. But the older child, because he took people's approval as a sign that he could do well, thought he had exceptional intelligence, and from an early age began working for a professional degree. Meanwhile, the younger one had little confidence, considered his brother brighter than he, and quit school at an early age to become a garage mechanic. Early rejection by others encourages self-rejection, and, in turn, neurosis. Most children tend (foolishly!) to accept themselves just about as much as they think others do.

Criticism. Children almost always take criticism as disapproval. Parents who continually nag a child indirectly say: "I see no good in you at all; in fact, you seem pretty hopeless" —even though they criticize for the child's "own good," even though they feel criticism necessary for teaching purposes, even though they have some justification for their criticism, no matter. To the child it indicates a lack of approval, a feeling of no-goodness. Whereupon he or she usually begins to believe in and profoundly feel this no-goodness.

The mother of one of my young female patients would say to her daughter: "Oh, you do the dishes badly." Or "Here, let me boil that egg. You'll only ruin it." Or "You go do your homework; I'll iron that dress for you." The mother thought this helped. Actually, it hindered enormously, for the daughter concluded that she could not, of herself, do anything correctly, that she had no good traits.

Perfectionism. If you teach a child to act perfectionistically you subtly and drastically criticize. For perfection does not exist, and excessive striving for it leads to disillusionment, heartache, and self-hatred. Perfectionists *must* act well or outstandingly at all times—which, of course, nobody will. You might just as well put a rope around a child's neck and tie a wild horse to the other end as try to instill in him or her a need for perfection.

Speaking of perfectionism recalls to mind another of my clients. She had such remarkable good looks that, at seventeen, when she first visited me, almost all the males in my waiting room immediately sat up and took notice. She had a tested Intelligence Quotient of 178 (a score obtained by about one out of a thousand individuals) and she had remarkable talents in dance and sculpting. But she thought herself ugly, stupid, and untalented. Why? Because from her earliest school years, whenever she came home with 97 or 98 in some subject, her mother, thoroughly unimpressed, would immediately complain: "So! And why couldn't you get 100?" As a result of taking this nonsense seriously (which children don't have to do but usually will), she had such a low estimate of herself that previous therapists labeled her "borderline psychotic."

Another client whose parents pointedly would associate only with the "best" people obtained fabulously good grades in all his college subjects—except art. Not only did he draw and paint very poorly, he even seemed unable to appreciate artistic masterpieces. This bothered him, and he took one art course after another to prove to himself that he could succeed at them. And whenever he received, as he invariably did, a mediocre grade, he disturbed himself. He insisted that he should do well in *everything*, and that he had something wrong with him if he did not. I had a hard time getting him to adopt a more realistic attitude.

Competitiveness. In our culture perfectionism often takes the form of extreme competitiveness. We teach children that they should do *better* than other children and should grow up to gain *greater* success. Statistically, of course, this won't work, since only a few outstanding individuals can actually perform consistently better than their fellows. The inevitable result: millions of Americans try frantically to keep up with the Joneses, or the champions, or the millionaires, and many of them end up feeling inadequate and depressed.

"Why," I ask my friends, relatives, and patients, "why must you do *better* than this person or that one?"

"Well, I just feel like a louse if I do not."

"But what makes you feel like a louse? How does it make you a *rotten person* if you don't do better than someone else?"

"I don't know. I just feel that way."

"But *why* do you feel that way?"

"I really can't say. I guess I haven't ever thought about the reason."

"Exactly! You have merely *accepted* the notion without thinking about it. Someone taught you to believe that doing better than someone else has advantages, and sometimes it does. But you escalate that into: 'I have worth for doing well.' You thereby foolishly overgeneralize: for your you-ness, your essence, you cannot legitimately rate. *You* have too much complexity, too much on-goingness to have a valid global rating."

This I say to my friends, relatives, and clients. Sometimes it does some good.

Unnecessary taboos. One of the main reasons people feel insecure involves their feeling guilty—because they think they have done something wrong or wicked, and damn themselves for doing it. Thus, the more things they deem wrong, the more taboos they have, the guiltier and more overwhelmed with feelings of inadequacy they feel. Our society carries on innumerable sexual, social, racial, religious, and other taboos some of which once had a rationale, but which today have outlived their usefulness. As a result, hordes of our citizens make themselves feel inordinately guilty and self-hating.

Take, by way of illustration, one of my acquaintances.

(I shall call him Mr. Potter.) Mr. Potter had very "good," strict parents. From early childhood they taught him that he should not play roughly or engage in any kind of sex play whatever, or talk back to his elders, or have a good time when any kind of work remained undone.

Mr. Potter had a list of don'ts in his early life thick enough to choke a human. It did. When I met him, in his thirtieth year, he had done miserably in his business, behaved impotently with his wife, and acted tyrannically with his son and daughter. The taboos with which he had gotten raised helped him feel like a villain when he didn't adhere to them closely and like a sissy when he did.

On both counts Mr. Potter felt inadequate. He acted as constrictedly as any individual I ever met, having narrowed down his positive enjoyments to subzero proportions and having replaced them with neurotic symptoms.

Sigmund Freud, one of the greatest psychologists, clearly saw the effects of unnecessary taboos on people. Unfortunately, prejudiced by the special sex taboos of the middle-class Viennese of the 1890s, Freud overemphasized the sexual aspects of neurosis, and at times implied that sex guilt created all inadequacy feelings. This, especially when applied to today, appears an overstatement. Freud, however, rightly stressed that *some* kind of taboo contributes to much of our guilt feelings; and that these feelings of guilt, in their turn, underly much of our emotional perplexity.

Spoiling. Overprotecting children helps destroy acceptance, too. For children who have everything done for them may grow up to believe that things *should* happen this way, and may never attempt to do anything for themselves. Or they may simply get no practice in taking chances, experimenting, or putting their ideas into action, and consequently will do so ineptly. When they finally discover the roughness of the world, they feel incapable of coping with it and begin to experience deep-seated feelings of inferiority.

Getting along well, like virtually all aspects of living, requires learning, practice, and effort. If, by the time you reach your teens and begin to think independently, you have had little previous experience in making decisions, you naturally find the going rough. This compares favorably to what would happen if, say, you tried at the age of sixteen to play baseball when in your entire previous life you had never thrown a ball or any other object.

To make matters even worse, you see other people, who seem to have had little experience and practice (but who actually have had much of both), do things routinely and automatically. Without any great difficulty, they ease their way over paths that appear strewn with unconquerable hurdles. Then, if you have gotten coddled and overprotected as a child, you falsely say to yourself, "Why can't I do things that well, that easily? What's happened to *me*?" You then, of course, experience even more intense feelings of inferiority.

An extreme example of this condition: the case of a man, who, at one and the same time, had gotten overprotected *and* rejected, spoiled *and* disapproved of by his parents during his childhood. When I saw him, at the age of forty, he refused, after literally thirty-five years of schooling, to accept a job as an assistant professor of English literature, although theoretically quite qualified.

This man's father had thoroughly rejected him, wanted him to act as a sportsman instead of a scholar, and never failed to criticize him for behaving as the father thought he shouldn't. To make matters worse, while criticizing the son, he continually bribed the boy with money and presents, so that he got what he wanted without working for anything.

The son chose to doubly dislike himself—because his father despised him and because he knew that he accepted his father's bribes without attempting to do anything for himself. And, since he had never really buckled down to doing anything difficult, at the age of forty he still lacked the experience that would ultimately make such difficult tasks easy. Hence, he refused to accept the professorial job for which he qualified.

Spoiling may encourage two major types of disordered emotions: self-hatred and an inability to tolerate frustration. Victims may down themselves or may refuse to accept the common frustrations of everyday living and make themselves overly irritable and hostile. Parental refusal to teach them to accept some of the grim realities of life may contribute much harm.

Frustration. Just as giving children everything they want may spoil them and encourage avoidance of life's responsibilities, unduly frustrating them may also encourage their acquiring a negative, unrealistic attitude. Humans, even though they can tolerate huge amounts of frustration, do have a breaking point. Young children particularly think they cannot stand the kind of frustrations imposed by overly rigid parents. You can force them into activities they loathe, but they may then make themselves feel serious resentment.

One of my former secretaries, the youngest of thirteen children, had a father who worked steadily but who never made enough money to satisfy the material needs of his large family. The mother did her best for all the children, but they still lacked many things. My secretary never had the toys, clothes, spending money, leisure, or other advantages that the other children in her neighborhood had. Very little of what she wanted did she ever get.

This woman grew up feeling unloved. She believed that life treated her and her family unfairly, and she felt little enthusiasm for living. Instead of trying to work harder (the logical thing to do in view of the family's economic needs), she gave up, viewed the situation as hopeless, and spent by far the greater part of her time bewailing her fate instead of trying to better it.

One of my clients lived as the only child in a well-to-do home. But his parents, who themselves came up through life the hard way, did not believe in earthly pleasures. They leaned over backward not to spoil their child—gave him virtually no toys, provided him with only a niggardly allowance, and opposed most of his plans for amusement. This man, too, almost exactly like the woman from the very poor family, felt so frustrated that he hardly knew which way to turn. He finally gave up trying, sabotaged his parents' desires for his success in life by refusing to work at anything, and failed miserably, first at school and then at a series of mediocre jobs. He could not see why, in view of the lack of earthly rewards for "good" behavior, he should work his head off for "nothing." So he organized a self-imposed emotional sit-down strike, refused to do anything he didn't have to do—and thereby, of course, hurt himself as well as his parents.

Suppressed hostility. A kind of frustration that many individuals think they cannot stand arises when they hate someone but feel constrained to suppress their hostility. Such suppressed anger often leads to internal simmering and seething, a transference of hatred to others, or a final, violent outburst of the suppressed feelings.

A young psychologist whom I supervised frothed and fumed because the head of the institution where he worked unduly restricted his activities. Powerless to do anything about this situation, the young man tended to act aggressively toward the inmates of the institution. When his superior warned him against this kind of aggression, he went on a wild driving spree one day, punched a policeman who arrested him for speeding, and wound up in the county jail. Fortunately, the judge before whom he appeared had himself had psychotherapy. He placed the psychologist on probation, with the proviso that he receive treatment.

Interestingly, when this psychologist did receive help, he functioned quite effectively in the same institution and under the same restrictive conditions that he had previously found so upsetting. For he then took the attitude that the administrator had emotional difficulties himself and therefore acted so tyrannically. Accepting this, the young psychologist refused any longer to make himself angry and to feel he had to displace his anger at his superior with aggression against the inmates.

In many important ways our society tends to encourage us to think unrealistically and to develop feelings of inadequacy and resentment. Then we damn ourselves so severely for feeling inadequate or hostile that we often erect neurotic defenses against admitting these faults. In turn, our defenses prevent us from tackling the irrational ideas behind our difficulties and doing something constructive about them.

Most neurosis seems to consist of irrational or exaggerated fear—which we generally call anxiety. Rational fear or concern occurs when you perceive real danger, as in fearing to cross a busy street without looking both ways. Irrational fright, overconcern, or anxiety, the fear you have when you exaggerate or invent danger, leads you to fear strolling on the sidewalk because you think a car might mount the curb and hit you.

People commonly fear physical injury and social disapproval. In comparison to primitive days, life today offers fewer chances of physical injury, for modern medical science, police forces, and protective devices have minimized such dangers. On the other hand, recent developments in atomic science and its war potential have sparked the growth of new physical fears.

The second prevalent human fear, that of social disapproval, may have increased with the years, since in some ways we now have more needs for conformity, for behaving like others, for keeping up with the Joneses, than our forefathers had. We often rear our children to think that getting love or approval has enormous value and that striving for self-acceptance has less virtue.

We teach the need for social approval in the family setting. As soon as children do anything wrong—anything the parents disapprove of or find inconvenient—their father or mother tends to pounce and say, "Don't do that, dear. If you do that *people won't love you.*" Or ". . . *nobody will like you.*" These phrases, usually said in a threatening tone and often backed up with a reproving slap or gesture, help children think it feels *terrible, horrible, awful,* if people—and especially parents—do not like them. They then tend to retain this early acquired belief, and never to question it in any way.

We also raise our children to blame themselves in many ways, particularly for their socially disapproved behavior. We give them a literature, from fairy tales to TV shows, replete with villains, "bad men," and wicked witches. We teach them to hate, to blame these villains, and to loathe themselves when they act "villainously."

Actually, of course, we cannot accurately label anyone "a villain" or "a louse" for several reasons:

1. "A villain" would behave *totally* villainously and could *only* and *always* act badly. How could we ever prove this?

2. Even if a person invariably performed villainously up to now, how could we know with any certainty that this dyed-in-the-wool "villain" would have a perfectly evil *future?*

3. "A villain" or "a louse" not only means a person who acts badly but one who has total responsibility and who therefore deserves severe punishment or eternal damnation

for acting so. But a person who consistently acts poorly has either hereditary and/or environmentally acquired tendencies to behave that way; and how has he or she total responsibility (much less damnability) for traits which he or she inherited or learned?

4. Even if a human has *total* free will or responsibility for his or her bad acts (which seems most unlikely), labeling that person as "a villain" or "a louse" clearly implies the existence of an immutable law of God or the universe that therefore he or she *deserves* or *should have* damnation for such acts. Where does the evidence for this law exist?

Because of an adherence to ancient views formulated long before we had any modern psychological knowledge, society still holds humans totally responsible for their crimes and demands that they down themselves and atone for their sins through punishment. And we demand this not only of external "villains" but of ourselves when we do wrong things.

Such a punitive philosophy makes us enormously guilty (rather than sincerely sorry) about many of the things we do; and guilt represents feelings of inadequacy or self-hatred. We do not contend that people should never feel responsible for their behavior. Whenever they needlessly, gratuitously, and willfully harm other humans, they'd better fully acknowledge their wrongdoing. But, even then, they'd better feel "guilty" only in the sense of resolving to make restitution and to avoid such actions again, and not in the sense of resolving to damn or punish themselves.

In other words, you can handle "guilt" in two ways—one rational and legitimate, and the other not. Rationally, acknowledge your wrongdoing or immorality. Thus, if you needlessly harm another (as by stealing from or physically hurting him or her), acknowledge your guilt—your responsibility for the act. Say to yourself: "Yes, I committed that offense. I behaved wrongly."

75

Irrationally, you can deal with "guilt" by going on from there and saying to yourself: "I *should not* have done that wicked deed. Only a villain would have done it. I have behaved unforgivably, and I deserve damnation and punishment."

We label this reaction irrational because, first of all, you foolishly tell yourself that you *should not or must not* have committed a wicked deed when, quite obviously, you *did.* You really mean: "I *would prefer* not to have committed the deed." Doubtless you would! But changing the sentence "I *would prefer* not to have done this" into "I *should not* have done it" makes no real sense. It posits some immutable law that states that you *must* not act immorally, and if such a law truly existed, you *could not* act so. When, moreover, can you ever prove any *must,* any guarantee, any absolute?

Secondly, telling yourself "Only a villain would have behaved so badly, and I should get punished for behaving villainously" implies that punishment will do some good—will help right the wrong done—and will help prevent you from harming someone again. Actually, no matter how you punish yourself, the person you harm reaps little benefit. And the whole history of human punishment shows that damning and punishing people for their sins does not effectively prevent them from doing evil things again. In fact, in some instances, when they label themselves rotten villains for doing rotten deeds, they assume that they *have* to act badly in the future (for that seems the nature of a villain)—and they compulsively do more bad deeds. Damnation and punishment do not improve people's acts because they induce them to bemoan their *past* deeds rather than to concentrate on how to change them *in the future.* If you tell yourself repeatedly "Oh, what a villain! I hurt John!," can you focus on the real problem: "How can I avoid hurting John (and others) in the future?" Not very well!

76

What can you do instead? Make the rational and legitimate observation: "I harmed John and I wrongly did so." Then, instead of irrationally continuing, "I must label myself a villain who deserves punishment for this deed," continue with "Granted that I did wrong this time, how can I make amends to John for my misdeeds, and how, especially, can I prevent myself from harming John again *next time?*"

If you take this tack, if you focus on how to *change* your poor behavior in the future instead of how to punish yourself for past misdeeds, you will increase your chances of figuring out a way to behave less immorally. But if you focus on self-condemnation and punishment, you will almost inevitably miss the real point—*learning* from your wrongdoings—and will continue to perpetrate them indefinitely.

The basis of rational morality, in other words, lies in two main propositions: First, if you needlessly harm others, these others or their associates will probably retaliate in kind, and you will tend to create a rather chaotic, frightful world for all of us to live in. Second, if you unnecessarily hurt someone, you'd better acknowledge your antisocial behavior and set about *changing* it for the better.

Unfortunately, however, most moralists have changed these two propositions into a significantly different form, and have contended that when you harm another, you flout some "natural" or "necessary" law of God and man, and you should mercilessly condemn and punish yourself and suffer damnation from others.

Actually, we do not necessarily act immorally when we harm someone else—for the good reason that we often find it *necessary* to harm another in order to survive ourselves. Thus, if you take a seat in a crowded train or make a profit on selling a house, you may benefit at the expense of others. But as long as you do not needlessly, deliberately, go out of your way to harm them, you do not act immorally. If you really do act

77

vilely toward another, beating yourself over the head will hardly right the wrong you have done. Sensibly resolve, in the present and in the future, to help the person you have harmed—or at least to refrain from harming him again.

Self-downing, then, results in neurosis-producing feelings of inadequacy. It accomplishes little to right any evil you have done. On the contrary, it generally prevents you from correcting your wrongs—and thereby encourages further self-blame. Positive, constructive regard for the present and future brings a logical solution to the problem of moral behavior. But our concepts of "villainy" and punishment sabotage such a solution.

In the last analysis neurosis stems from a moral problem, and Sigmund Freud saw correctly when he viewed it as a conflict between what he called the superego (or conscience) and people's unconscious strivings (the id), on the one hand, and their conscious desires (the ego), on the other. Freud, however, made too much of people's sex drives and conflicts and too little of their nonsexual impulses.

When people label certain aspects of their behavior as wrong or wicked, and when, instead of doing something constructive about changing these activities, they berate themselves for continuing to perform them, they end up by hating themselves. This self-loathing leads them to various other neurotic symptoms such as inertia, goofing, alcoholism, and overeating. Then, in turn, their very neurotic traits encourage them to hate themselves still more, and to behave more neurotically. Here we have a circle that, in terms of the construction and maintenance of a healthy, productive, happy personality, we can call not only vicious but positively lethal!

5

How to Help a "Neurotic" Overcome Disturbance

You can best live with "neurotics" by helping them overcome their neuroses. Have you this possibility? Can people with disturbances actually get better? Find effective "cures"? Categorically, yes. But not easily!

"Neurotics" can overcome disturbance, and get help from another person because the disturbance stems from irrational, unrealistic ideas they largely teach themselves, and which (with some difficulty) they can unlearn or change. Neurotic symptoms such as feelings of anxiety, rage, guilt, and depression follow crooked thinking. You can consequently help those afflicted with these symptoms by encouraging them to change their beliefs.

People with irrational thinking leading to neurosis largely hold it unconsciously, but do not, as the orthodox Freudians believe, so deeply hide and repress it that they cannot bring it to consciousness without a long psychoanalytic process. They can bring to the surface their irrational ideas—for instance, "I must act competently!"—by inferring them from their disordered behavior. The gap between their rational conscious beliefs and their disturbed behavior indicates their irrational unconscious beliefs.

Once "neurotics" see that they have some fundamental irrational beliefs, you can help them attack these beliefs by pointing up their silliness, by inducing them to act against these beliefs, and by other techniques described in this chapter. You may find this difficult, but still quite possible.

You cannot easily help change "neurotics" because frequently they do not wish to admit, in the first place, that they have emotional problems. And, even when they do, they often refuse outside aid, and insist that they will help themselves. Sometimes when they do want help, they unconsciously resist it because they so accustom themselves to their own symptoms that they see them vaguely or inaccurately. And sometimes they resist help because they feel so ashamed of their neurotic behavior that they have difficulty facing it.

Neurotic habits have two edges: they spring from some irrational idea; and they embody that idea in some inappropriate practice. To overcome such habits, you work on both the underlying idea and the practice. A boy, for example, stutters because he fears speaking badly in front of other people. But even if he gets over this fear of speaking poorly, he still has the motor habit of stuttering (perhaps of many years' standing) to overcome. Naturally, he has trouble doing this.

If you squelch a neurotic habit without getting at its underlying cause, you may replace it by another equally obnoxious habit. Thus, if you stutter because you fear that you will utter nasty words, and you merely work on the habit of stuttering, you may overcome that habit but still feel anxious about saying nasty words. In such a case, you may develop some other neurotic symptom, such as attacks of colitis or a fear of going visiting. For this reason, many therapists feel reluctant to use hypnosis, simple reassurance, drugs, penalties, and certain other techniques that sometimes help your habit or symptom without getting at the root of your neurosis and changing your basic personality pattern.

Neurosis consists of disordered emotions and/or defensive behavior that may prevent you from consciously facing your disturbed feelings. To conquer a neurosis, you'd better understand it and attack the ideas behind it, and also work through the habits that comprise it. Occasionally, insight into the causes of your symptoms quickly and automatically leads to clearing them up. Much more often, however, insight merely lays the groundwork for changing your ideas and undoing your symptoms. Their actual eradication calls for much further work—and *work* alone, usually, will get the job done.

Relatives and friends may in particular aid "neurotics" because unlike a psychotherapist who sees his clients an hour or two each week, they see them continuously, and, by their own attitudes toward disturbance, they can help reduce it. In my own therapeutic work I frequently use my clients' associates as auxiliary therapists and sometimes find that I can succeed better through their efforts than by means of my own. This particularly goes for young children, whom I treat largely by working with their parents. But it also goes for many so-called adults.

Trying to help "neurotics" has difficulties because it requires several traits and some knowledge not too commonly found in the average person. For example, you'd better not behave too neurotically yourself. If so, you will tend to have so many problems of your own and have so little objectivity that you can hardly aid anyone else. You'd do well to have considerable patience and energy to devote to the task of helping "neurotics." Also of great help: keen insight into human behavior and understanding of both yourself and others. Again, don't expect to treat disturbed friends and relatives as a therapist would treat clients, because your relationship to them usually has much more personal involvement than does the relationship of a professional therapist to those she or he treats.

Your first step toward helping people behave less neurotically? Recognize clearly and *accept* the fact that they have disturbances. Many of us who have rather disturbed relatives or friends simply refuse to accept the fact that these people behave unusually and continue to treat them as if they had perfect adjustment. "Neurotics" do not act like adjusted adults. And if you treat them as if they can easily live up to the kinds of behavior expected of non-"neurotics," they will quickly disappoint you. Then, if you show your displeasure, they will often feel they have failed—hence, they will tend to make themselves more neurotic.

You may not readily accept "neurotics'" emotional disturbances. As explained in the first chapter, they often act unreliably, angrily, ungratefully, egoistically, and unlovingly. Trying to accept them with their undesirable traits seems like trying to live with a blackguard or an enemy. But, if you want to help them, you'd better accept them almost without reservation.

Of course, you do not *have* to accept a "neurotic," even a close relative like a sister or a husband. Except for children you voluntarily bring into the world (and in consequence have a moral duty to help), you *need* not help anyone. But if, because of emotional or other ties, you do wish to help, you'd better *fully* accept a "neurotic."

This means that as soon as your relatives or associates do something particularly stupid, pigheaded, or irritating, you can ask yourself: "*Why* did they do that?" And quickly answer: "Because of their neuroses! Because 'neurotics' frequently, usually, do that sort of thing. Not because they hate me. Not because they personally aim to do me in. Because

82

they often behave neurotically. And 'neurotics' commonly do vicious, stupid, ruthless things."

In other words, don't respond to "neurotics'" actions as if they direct them personally and specifically against you. And even when they do, you can realize that these anti-you actions, the result of neurosis, often stem from anti-self feelings. Pity them for feeling so disturbed, for seeming compelled to act in a sometimes vicious manner. But do not *damn* them for acting thus.

Remember that "neurotics" rarely deliberately choose their obnoxious behavior. They partly inherit and they partly acquire a strong tendency to act neurotically. They do not *wish* to feel emotionally upset; do not voluntarily select the path to neurosis. They mainly hate themselves. Even when they harm others, they virtually compel themselves to do this harm by their irrational views.

Whom, then, can we blame for an individual's neurosis, if he or she does not have complete responsibility? His other parents or grandparents? Hardly. For they, too, behaved disturbedly or ignorantly, and did not know what they did. Can we blame society? In a way, yes—since it produced all of us. Actually, though, society consists of people, and if people happen to have limitations and ignorance, and if they unwittingly construct and perpetuate foolish laws and customs, should we rightfully condemn them?

Why, indeed, damn anyone? Certainly, this set of factors may cause that set of conditions. But will damning people stop the set of factors from operating or prevent it from leading to a consequent set of conditions? Let us ask: How can we *change* these factors and *prevent* these conditions from occurring? Why not concentrate on this question instead of on the question of whom we must condemn?

To repeat, take the first step to help a "neurotic" by accepting, fully, the fact that he or she acts disturbedly and by resisting damning him or her in any way for acting so.

Once you face the fact that a parent. child, sibling, mate, friend, or business associate has a serious neurosis, you can next understand what "neurotics" do, why they behave the way they behave, and how you can help them change. You will find material useful for that understanding in the pages of this book. Other valuable material you will find in the newer works on psychotherapy and personality theory, a selected list of which appears in the last chapter. Read some of this material. Attend seminars, workshops, and lectures on personality and human behavior given by local universities, therapy institutes, and growth centers (such as the Institute for Advanced Study in Rational Psychotherapy in New York City). Keep well informed on psychological findings. The more you learn about psychology in general, and psychotherapy in particular, the better you can understand yourself and help others with their problems.

Your *self*-understanding has special importance in the comprehension of the emotional quirks of others. Anything you do to look into your own heart, discover your own neurotic leanings, and remedy your emotional blockings will tend to help you help others.

Although you may not feel too seriously disturbed, one of the best things you can do, if you have difficulty helping a neurotic relative or friend, includes having some amount of consultation or aid yourself. Remember in this connection, in addition to helping people to overcome their emotional problems, a major therapy goal involves showing reasonably nondisturbed or midly neurotic individuals how to understand themselves and to conquer those irrationalities that prevent them from achieving their maximum potential.

Once you stand ready to fully accept "neurotics" and to learn enough about psychology to understand them, your next step can include giving warmth and support. For we cannot too often emphasize that "neurotics" employ self-downing —foolishly believe that *they* have no value when their *performances* fail and others disapprove of them. They can more easily accept themselves, therefore, if you unconditionally accept *them* in spite of their poor *deeds*.

"Neurotics," alas, often do not seem to deserve any acceptance or warmth. Instead, they frequently go out of their way to bring on rejection and disapproval. They often view with suspicion almost any kindness shown them and test out their friends with ungrateful, negative responses. Consequently, they demand consistent, unvarying love, and continue to demand it before they begin to believe that you really feel it for them.

This does not mean that you should shamelessly flatter "neurotics" in an effort to build up their ego-strength. On the contrary, they may quickly see behind such flattery and it will boomerang. Rather, bolster them intelligently, with as much truth as possible. Bring their good points to their attention; show them how they perform effectively at this or that—however ineptly they may do something else.

In other words, emphasize their assets. Do not falsely deny their failings, but try to ignore or minimize them. Keep bringing up their good points at appropriate moments. Let them know when they look especially good, when they do a fine job, when they act better than they thought they could. Don't emphasize their assets only in words, but also by your *attitudes*. Take the attitude that you need not rate any humans, including your neurotic associates, as good or bad people, but can accept them as people who do good and bad acts. Really convince yourself of this so that you will communicate your attitude to "neurotics" you would help.

Above all, encourage them to do the things they foolishly fear and erroneously believe they cannot do successfully. Encourage their efforts, even though they may fail. And if they do fail, show them that the next attempt may well succeed. Try to induce "neurotics" to do things at which they will probably succeed. Then point out that these successes indicate that they can do other things that they fear.

Convince your neurotic friends or relatives that everyone frequently fails and that humans mainly learn by trial and error. Therefore, failure not only commonly occurs, but has great advantages. We learn by it and thereby help ourselves to succeed in the future.

Sometimes help "neurotics" lower their level of aspiration so that they don't attempt things beyond their ability. Encourage them to act daringly—but realistically. Discourage perfectionism or highly unrealistic expectations.

You can also help "neurotics" see that though success may have importance, *you* do not see it as all-important or sacred. Show confidence in their future success, but when they fail, show that you still accept and care for them.

In showing "neurotics" that you wholeheartedly respect them as humans, simultaneously make it clear that you cannot permit them to see you as an easy mark for exploitation or abuse. Adopt an attitude of firm kindness and avoid pampering and babying them.

What do I mean by *firm kindness?* Just what it implies. It means you act nicely to people, but set definite limits as to how far they may impose on you and firmly stick to those limits. It means your seeing things from other people's frames of reference, but never entirely losing sight of your own vital wants and interests.

Suppose, for example, you have a neurotic husband who fears meeting people, and wants to sit home every night and never have any visitors. Don't say "Now look here, Joe, you know feeling afraid of people means you have great neurotic stupidity. Besides, you have no consideration for me. You never think of what *I* want to do. If you really loved me, you'd get over your silly notions, take me out regularly, and feel pleased when I ask people in."

That kind of talk will help convince Joe that he possesses total inadequacy, that you just do not understand him, and that you think only of yourself. It will encourage him to feel more disturbed.

As Joe's wife, you'd better realize that his refusal to see people results from neurotic anxiety and self-downing. Do everything possible to help him feel that he *can* get along with people. Work at perhaps gradually getting him to meet one or two compatible people at first—preferably people you have alerted to his problems, so that they will accept him. Once he feels somewhat at ease with these new friends, you can help him realize that he can get along with other people as well.

If, however, Joe remains stubbornly neurotic about meeting people and insists that you stay at home too, you may say something like this: "I really understand, Joe, that you don't want to meet people right now, though I feel you will want to later on. In the meantime, I shall nearly go crazy, steadily cooped up like this. I really want to see people now and then. I don't mind your not wanting them, but I have no intention of feeling the same. Now, suppose I stay home with you most of the time, but every once in a while go out by myself. Then, when you get over not wanting to. see people, which I think you will, we can have a fine time going out together."

Working along these lines, you can stand up for your own rights and, at the same time, show an understanding of other people's neuroses. To let your neurotic mate run you completely, merely because of his disturbance, often gives him an incentive to prolong or intensify it. For he then has an excuse to act like a baby, expecting to get his own way.

Moreover, he may lose respect for you and put himself down for associating with someone as weak and namby-pamby as you.

Besides, "neurotics" often do not really completely want their own way. They want understanding, acceptance, and approval. Frequently, they know they behave incorrectly and feel worse because no one stops them. One of my own relatives, for example, enjoyed her husband's concessions when she made unreasonable demands. But when he let her spend all their vacation money for a trip by herself, while he stayed home in the sweltering city, she loathed his weakness and hated her taking advantage of him. These feelings served to increase her disturbance.

"Neurotics" want, sometimes more than anything else, someone they can see as a good model, with whom they can identify, and from whom they can gain strength. They even undertake psychotherapy for this purpose—not merely to gain love and understanding from their therapists, but to use their strength, their personality, their non-neurotic behavior. I met with this situation when a client, referred to me and to another therapist, obtained interviews with both of us and then decided to stay with me. "What made you decide against the other man and in my favor?" I asked.

"Well, as it happened," my client replied, "I went to see him, and I first noticed his room filled with smoke. I want to cut down on my smoking. Then, he spoke in a low tone of voice that I could hardly hear. Finally, I saw that he weighed about 250 pounds. And, as I told you last time, I have a weight problem. Well, I said to myself, if he has such poor discipline in his own life, I don't see how he could possibly help me very much!"

The stronger and less indecisively you act, the more "neurotics" will probably trust you, and feel confident that you can help them. So, act firmly with them. You'd also better decide on the limits of attention you will give to them, and then adhere to these limits. Treat them kindly *and* firmly, not one *or* the other.

Don't permit a person you seek to help to blackmail you emotionally. Frequently, as in the case of mothers who suddenly acquire a heart condition or severe indigestion just when their favorite son's wedding approaches, "neurotics" use sickness for blackmailing purposes. If able to get others to do things their way by pleading illness or acute unhappiness, they sometimes turn into chronic sufferers and continue to exploit you unmercifully. Don't submit to this kind of blackmail, for "neurotics" can behave very much like martyrs. Act kindly but stand firm.

One central rule in dealing with a "neurotic": *do not criticize!* As we have pointed out previously, "neurotics" arrive at their state largely from taking criticism too seriously. Because they make themselves oversensitized, they take further criticism badly. If you down them (or even their traits), you may contribute to increasing their feelings of worthlessness.

Criticism, moreover, rarely moves people to constructive action. Helping humans to change their "poor" behavior for "better" behavior involves inducing them to go from point 1 to point 2. But most of us, when told that we *should* move from 1 to 2 or that we behave like idiots for not so moving, balk or go backward. We resent any pushing or pressuring even for our own good.

"Neurotics," in particular, tend to react poorly to appeals that take the form of criticism. To tell them that they should, for their own good, go from point 1 to 2 equals: "Look here, you fool! You know darned well that you harm yourself by remaining at 1 instead of going to 2. Now why don't you stop acting like a dunce and do the right thing?" To almost anyone this will sound like censure.

"Neurotics" constantly blame themselves for behaving "crazily," for having disturbed symptoms; and if you condemn them, this only helps increase their self-damning. You can, instead, *not* attack them or even their behavior, but the *ideas* that lie behind their symptoms. If, for example, your neurotic friend fears riding on trains, don't tell him: "Oh, come on, Jim. How silly! You know that trains have a safe record!" Certainly he knows how silly his phobia sounds and that riding in trains involves no great danger. But if you emphasize these irrationalities, you label him as an idiot. Instead, try to find the idea behind Jim's fear of riding in trains. Obviously, he believes riding in trains involves great danger. Thus, he may have thoughts that the train will crash, and that would mean utter disaster. Or, that in a crowded train he has to have close physical contact with a man or woman, and he views that as unbearable. Or, that if he had an attack of diarrhea in a train he might not get to the bathroom in time, and that would seem most embarrassing. If you want to undermine Jim's phobia, you'd better discover what irrational ideas Jim dreams up to create his anxiety, and then tackle not Jim, and not even his anxiety, but his irrational ideas.

Thus, if you discover that Jim really fears dying in a train crash, you could point out that very few crashes occur these days; that most of those that do occur result in few fatalities; that everyone has to die someday; that worrying about the possibility of a train crash will hardly reduce the chances of a train's actually crashing; that preserving his life at the expense of continual worry (and avoiding trains) hardly seems worth the effort; and so on.

This type of attack on the ideological bases of "neurotics'" fears will often do a lot of good. In many instances, however, just because you have intimate relations with them, they expect certain things that they ordinarily would not expect from others. In such cases, you get called upon to do something more to overcome their inertia and to induce them to move from a harmful to a beneficial point. What more?

The answer, in large part, includes love. Out of love for another, a person will not only move in a desired direction but will actually endure injury or even death if it would help the other. If you really convince "neurotics" that you care, that you see things from their frame of reference, they will often do virtually anything for you, including, at times, surrendering some neurotic behavior.

Consider the problem of a man who wants to have frequent sex with his wife. But the wife, because of a neurotic fear of too-frequent activity, desires to have sex only once or twice a month. If he uses ridicule, she balks all the more. If he pleads, she says that she would like to have sex more often, but just can't feel comfortable having it. Impasse. The more he ridicules or pleads, the more uncomfortable she feels, and the more her neurosis intensifies.

The husband can try a different tack. He can understand his wife's predicament, show her that he realizes she has her reasons, and not accuse her of hostility. He can also try to discover the basic cause for her fear of sex and to show her that even though she once may have had good reasons for it, these no longer apply. He'd better not make fun of her sex fears or superstitions, but attempt to get behind and undermine them with different, more rational attitudes.

Above all, he can give her love and show her that in spite of his own disappointment, he does not resent her. Admitting frankly his inconvenience, he can try to get her to satisfy him in noncoital ways if she balks at intercourse. He can honestly show his own feelings, but at the same time show her that he loves her, even though he may not love the inconvenience she causes him.

If you consistently, wholeheartedly care for "neurotics" even when they inconvenience or deprive you, they will feel

that at least one person respects them, and may begin to surrender the feelings of inadequacy and hostility that underlie
neurosis. Secondly, they may feel that they have in you a
partner, a true helper, therefore a better chance to overcome
fears and disturbances. Thirdly, they will tend to love you in
return, and out of this love they will often begin, quite
spontaneously, to do things for you that they would not think
of doing for anyone else in the world—including, quite possibly, trying to overcome neurotic fears that inconvenience
you.

Love begets love; and begotten love often begets action.
This does not work invariably, since your spouse may behave
so neurotically about sex or other impulses that even extreme
love may not induce him or her to try to work through neurosis. But, as therapists have seen since Freud's day, clients
can gain insight and develop actions to complement that
insight through their positive feelings, or love, for a therapist.
Similarly, in a nontherapeutic relationship, if you can somehow induce "neurotics" to love you, they sometimes begin
to work on their own cure.

Your next important step in trying to help "neurotics"
can include doing something to relieve their shame or guilt.
At bottom, virtually all of them feel ashamed or guilty—fearful of doing the wrong things and that others will therefore
not like them. To relieve this, you can use two main procedures: relating in a lenient, noncritical, and permissive
fashion when they do something "bad" or mistaken; and encouraging them to conform to their own standards and to
do the things they consider right.

Consider, first, the policy of leniency. "Neurotics" tend
to allow themselves little leniency in many areas. They criticize themselves for every little wrong, and forgive themselves
little or nothing. If you, therefore, act permissively and for-
givingly, they may tend to accept themselves more.

Suppose you live with a man who feels guilty about not loving his mother sufficiently. If you act as if having ambivalent feelings toward one's mother hardly constitutes a crime, he may take a different attitude toward his own lack *EG* of love. Or, taking a somewhat different approach, you can try to discover why he dislikes his mother and help him overcome this dislike.

In expressing permissiveness with "neurotics," your own attitudes and actions may prove more important than your *modeling* words. If a woman feels enormously guilty about her sex activities, merely telling her not to feel guilty will hardly suffice if you have similar guilt and show it. As a guiltless model yourself, you have one of the best opportunities to reach her.

The other approach to reducing guilt—that of discouraging disturbed people from doing things they will make themselves feel guilty about—seems directly opposed to the first approach. But, no. For humans who live in any form of society had better feel wrong about some of the things they do, otherwise that society would not exist very long. If no one thought it wrong to steal, rape, or murder, everyone would try at times to get away with these acts, and chaos would result.

Although you can remain permissive and forgiving with "neurotics," don't try to take away their entire sense of wrongdoing, but only their unnecessary guilt. In terms of the philosophy outlined in the last chapter, try to induce them to think when they do something needlessly harmful to others, "I did this deed, and I see it as wrong. All right, admitting my wrong, now let me see how I can make restitution for this deed and stop myself from repeating it in the future." Not: "What a terrible villain I prove myself for committing this deed! Let me see how I can best damn and punish myself for doing it."

In getting "neurotics" to admit their mistaken or immoral behavior and to concentrate on not repeating it in the future, you can often help by inducing them to avoid the activities (or lack of activities) that led to their wrongdoing.

Suppose, for instance, that a man, in order to have sex, lies to a woman, saying that he wishes to marry her, when actually he has no desire to divorce his present wife. Under these conditions, he will tend to feel uncomfortable—as well he might. You can help reduce his guilt by inducing him to stop lying and to accept the consequences of telling the truth, even if this means that the woman will refuse to have anything more to do with him.

However, don't say to him, "Look here, Jack, how *awful* for you to treat the woman like that! Why don't you stop behaving like a louse and tell her the truth?" Such behavior will probably help increase his guilt, encourage his feeling that everyone hates him, and help him to find some rationalization for his behavior.

Instead, try to get this person to change his behavior by showing him that unless he does things the hard way, unless he lives a reasonably moral life, he himself will lose—since he will deny his *own* concepts of morality, and in the long run will gain more suffering than pleasure. Or, in other words, any satisfaction gained by engaging in behavior of which he, himself, disapproves will tend to bring on painful feelings of irresponsibility and immorality. And, in the final analysis, he gains less satisfaction than pain, even if he wisely refrains from downing himself.

Sometimes, by remaining calm yourself, by continuing to accept guilt-ridden people, and by showing interest in reducing instead of augmenting their feelings of guilt, you can show them how to stop feeling irrationally guilty or how to stop doing the things about which they'd better feel irresponsible and uncomfortable.

94

If people you try to help have done truly immoral or unwise things, you can try to get them to use their feelings constructively rather than destructively. For if they have made bad mistakes and have needlessly harmed others thereby, they'd still better not resort to self-condemnation. Their acknowledging wrongdoing can help prevent them from repeating the wrong behavior. It does not "prove" how they have no human worth for doing it.

Thus, if your son has unnecessarily harmed a neighbor's child, you can show him that he has acted improperly, and that the remedy for his antisocial behavior does not lie in his punishing himself (or in your punishing him), but in resolving to act better to the other child in the future. Or if your "neurotic" wife feels inordinately guilty because she has not taken care of the house properly, you can show her that she can first stop damning herself and then try to act as a more model housekeeper.

The main objective, then, when dealing with neurotic guilt, rests in convincing disturbed people that they really have nothing to feel guilty (self-downing) about, but that if they actually behaved badly they can remove their sense of immorality by trying to behave better. If you can implant this idea in guilt-burdened "neurotics," you may help them considerably.

One effective way of helping neurotic friends overcome feelings of guilt and worthlessness may include reducing certain demands on them, at least temporarily. Many troubled people, because they consume energy hating themselves and others, feel overburdened by the regular work of caring for a home, running a business, or participating in organizational activity. At times, they may display acute exhaustion, develop different kinds of physical symptoms, get extremely agitated, or even go into a severe state of depression.

If so, you would do well in many instances to reduce their load. Then, after you help them by means of some of the other methods discussed in this chapter, they can fully resume active responsibilities again.

In gauging the work load that "neurotics" can realistically maintain, take care, while not insisting that they do too much, not to permit them to do too little either. For work itself, especially when productive, can prove anti-neuroticizing.

Sometimes you can encourage more, rather than less, activity for disturbed individuals, since such activity may serve to divert them from their neurotic thinking. So, although temporarily they may have reduced responsibilities, in a few months you may arrange to have them increased again. If you carefully observe disturbed friends or relatives, and get them to experiment with different kinds of work responsibilities, you can ordinarily help them to work out schedules suitable to overcoming their self-flagellation. In deciding on a specific program, however, you may also require some professional consultation.

Clearly the biggest hurdle "neurotics" have to overcome they create by irrational fears: such as fear of rejection and of failure. Sometimes, one can reason with them, show the silliness of the fears, and bring them to a rational viewpoint. In so doing, however, you will find tackling the fears themselves often ineffective. Instead, ferret out and attack the irrational ideas behind the fears.

Thus, if your neurotic cousin fears playing tennis, little good will result from telling him, "You can enjoy this game. How silly not to try it!" He knows this already and probably hates himself—partly because he does know it.

Your cousin does not know that he has some underlying belief that makes tennis appear hazardous to him, when he really has no evidence of its dangerousness. Thus, he may believe that if he played tennis badly people would disapprove of him, and that he couldn't bear the "danger" of disapproval. This belief has no sensible foundation, since people would not disapprove of *him* but only of his *playing*. And if they did, he could definitely *bear* their disapproval and see it as not dangerous.

Rather than attack your cousin's fears directly, you can more effectively attack the irrational *ideas* that lie behind them and that force him, as long as he retains such ideas, to have the fears. You can undermine such fears, again, if you ferret them out, show your cousin that he has them, point out their illogical foundations, and demonstrate how they lead to trouble, and how he can dispute them.

You can attack irrational beliefs leading to needless fears by helping people get more familiar with the things they fear. By direct contact they will often overcome their fear of previously avoided things. Humans, in fact, find it hard to remain afraid of virtually anything when they have sufficient familiarity with it. High mountain peaks, bloody hand-to-hand battles, bleak ocean wastes—even these seem less frightening to most people who come into steady contact with them. Also, when they continue to practice some activity, people acquire more competence at it. And increasing competence helps drive away the greatest and most widespread of all our fears today—fear of failure.

Avoiding fear, moreover, reinforces or rewards it. If you run away from the things you find "dangerous," you keep yourself from getting familiar with these things or getting practice at them. By temporarily reducing your anxiety, you tend to make yourself more loath to face the thing you fear. You (and your neurotic friends) not only then remain irrationally afraid of something, but also refrain from doing the thing you fear, and wind up by increasing its "dangers."

You may employ a number of different techniques to

97

help "neurotics" face the things they fear. For example, you can serve as an excellent model by doing the feared act yourself and challenging its "terror." Or you can go along to keep them company in doing something they will not face alone, such as taking a plane ride. Occasionally you can trick them into doing some presumably awesome thing—getting them to take a first plane trip, perhaps, by pretending your car doesn't work, and that a plane remains the only practical means of transportation for the moment.

More frequently, you can induce disturbed people to challenge their fears by offering some special incentive—paying for a vacation trip if they will take a plane instead of a train or bus. Or you can sometimes help condition them to a feared experience by pairing it with a nonfeared or pleasant experience. The choice of paired activities would, of course, vary according to each individual case.

By fair means or foul, then, you can somehow induce your neurotic associates to keep doing things they fear, and they will then often lose their fears and may even start enjoying the "frightening" things. Nothing succeeds like success. If you can help people to survive contact with an irrationally feared person or thing, they will normally overcome their negative attitudes toward it.

Many years ago, before I even had the idea of practicing psychology, I befriended an exceptionally shy male, Roger, who wanted very much to succeed with women, but who rarely had the courage to ask them for dates or to make any moves toward them when he did occasionally date them. He acted so backwardly in this respect that he would know a female for months and never try to hold her hand or to kiss her good night.

I wanted to help Roger but didn't know exactly what I could do. So I enlisted the aid of my own steady woman, Roberta, a vivacious and very sociable person. She immediately tackled the problem and came up with what seemed to me a practical solution. I let Roberta know whenever I expected Roger to visit me, and she would arrange to come over, bringing with her one of her attractive and intelligent woman friends—fortunately, she had many of them. Then, after spending some time at my place, she would see to it that I walked home with her, leaving Roger, of course, with the other woman.

We tried this procedure several times and it soon began to take effect. Not only did we force Roger to see several females, but Roberta would subsequently manage to let him know that he had made a hit with this or that one, and that she would very much like to see him again. He soon began to feel at ease while talking to these women and, in addition, to believe that he could make a good impression on them.

After a while, Roger began to acquire an entirely different picture of his prowess, actually viewing himself as something of a captivating young man. Moved by this picture to act more daringly, he began to make affectionate overtures and to gain acceptance in a reasonable percentage of his tries. Before long, he started to see himself as a kind of young Casanova! The whole business ended when he started going steadily with one woman. Ultimately he married her—many years in fact before either my woman friend or I (we eventually parted) managed to maneuver ourselves into the state of matrimony!

"Neurotics" may sometimes get help from interpretations of the specific reasons for the continuance of their disturbances. But amateurs had better use this method with extreme caution! Even in the hands of a trained psychotherapist, detailed interpretations of the causes of neurosis often prove doubled-edged swords, requiring careful usage.

In making specific interpretations a conventional therapist generally says something like this: "Let us see, now. You say that you think your resentment toward your boss arises out of the inconsiderate way he treats you. Could you, however, fail to see the whole story? Could you actually hate your boss, at least in part, because he resembles your father, and because you transfer to him some of the old attitudes you had toward your father?"

Or the therapist may say: "According to the story you've told me, you seem, on the surface, to love your mother dearly and to feel sorry you've caused her all this heartache with your delinquent behavior. Your acts themselves, however, would seem to indicate that you do everything possible to help cause her the heartache that you say you want to prevent. Could you, unconsciously, really resent your mother and almost deliberately keep acting the way you do, because you realize that this would hurt her most?"

This kind of specific interpretation, relating the individual's conscious thinking and behavior to underlying, unconscious feelings, constitutes one of the important aspects of intensive psychotherapy or psychoanalysis. The therapist can make such interpretations because he has a wide knowledge of human personality, because he knows the particular client quite intimately, and because his training enables him to select a true and useful interpretation among many false and useless alternatives. Even then, the therapist often errs interpretively, and had better feel prepared to confess his mistakes and rectify them with better interpretations.

Because, as a friendly helper, you do not have the training to select accurate interpretations, and because you may more often than not err in making them, take great care about getting into this area of therapy when you attempt to help a "neurotic." Usually, if you do make interpretations, you had best make them only when good rapport exists between you and your neurotic associates. And you had best not attempt to cram them willy-nilly down their throats. Make interpretations, moreover, cautiously and tentatively, without dogmatism. Instead of saying, "Because you do this and think that, obviously this other thing must follow," say, "In view of the fact that you say and do this, do you possibly also do that?"

If you do not try to act as a psychoanalyst and do not project your own disturbances onto others, you may help a neurotic friend gain some valuable insights. If you stick to general rather than specific points, you will tend to stay on the safe side. Thus, you may safely assume that "neurotics" keep telling themselves that *something awful* or *terrible* may occur and thereby create their emotional hassles. But you may not easily discover *what* they feel awful about. Therefore, you can more safely try to help them discover, themselves, what "terrible" things they invent.

You may especially use general interpretations of this sort with individuals who avoid therapeutic help. Sometimes you may lead these people to a therapist by starting the interpretative ball rolling and then explaining that you do not have the training to go too far. But watch your step! No matter how gentle or cautious you may remain, you may go farther than your disturbed friends feel they can tolerate. If they grow defensive and resistant, or seem agitated or depressed, consult a professional psychotherapist before going any further.

You may more safely try to help "neurotics" by giving them advice and support. Almost by definition, most of them have trouble standing on their own two feet, and therefore seek others for advice. But what advice can you best give them? Quite a question!

In the main, stick to cooperative planning. For instance, instead of merely telling neurotic associates what to do (and practically doing it for them), plan *with* them and give them the feeling that they create most of the planning.

Otherwise they may take the best-meant advice as

101

criticism of their own inability to solve problems. Or they may accept your support so wholeheartedly that they make themselves utterly dependent on outside help. Giving "neurotics" the idea that they think and do *with* rather than *through* you tends to help them more effectively change their behavior.

You'd better time well your advice and support. The less people function for themselves, the more they can use your support. If they really cannot seem to work effectively, have confused ideas and feelings, act childishly, and keep getting into trouble, allowing dependency for a while may do a lot of good.

If your neurotic friends seem "spoiled," really able to do things for themselves, but demanding that others take over their lives, giving too much support may encourage dependency forever. Or, if they once felt helpless, but now feel stronger and ready to take their own steps, too much support can prove harmful. In general, try to give the degree of support and advice that "neurotics" seem to require at a given time, but don't overdo this bolstering to fulfill your own demands to have dependents.

Several years ago I treated a woman who appeared exceptionally disturbed, after her rejection by successive lovers. Wrongly, I tried to lead her, for a time, away from other intense emotional involvements in which she might hurt herself again. Whenever she told me about some new male she had met, I would encourage her to discover all possible information about him, and to take his initially favorable attitudes toward her very skeptically.

Things went quite well for a while, probably because she managed to avoid all harrowing involvements. But then, one day she seemed on the brink of the precipice again. She had met a "most fascinating" man and very soon felt intensely enamored of him. For his part, he seemed to reciprocate her feelings, but I remained skeptical. He had, it appeared, outstanding traits, and I wondered how much he would attach himself to my client, who, although quite charming, had such obvious disturbances.

I therefore did everything possible to help my client to put the brakes on her feelings for this new man and to question his attitudes toward her. To no avail. "I know for certain," she insisted, "that I do not delude myself with him as I did with those other fellows. And I know that I can take care of myself this time, even if the affair goes wrong."

"All right," I said, "but don't forget the risks involved."

"I'll willingly take them."

I couldn't do more. In spite of my misgivings, she continued with the affair. A few weeks later, my worst expectations seemed fulfilled. Her new boyfriend proved fickle, and she had difficulty discovering how he actually felt toward her. Much to my surprise, however, she handled the situation with unusual calmness and maturity, and not only refrained from hurting herself, but so impressed her boyfriend with her good sense and stability that his own doubts vanished. A few months later they married, and to my knowledge have remained happy. This case taught me a good lesson: not to underestimate an individual's power to overcome disturbance. If a "hurt" person refrains from later love risks, she may preserve her tendency to down herself about rejection—and may stay just as neurotic as ever.

You may often best help people with troubles by actions rather than words and by serving as a good model yourself. For they frequently copy the behavior of poor life models—particularly their parents. If you can serve as a better model, they will often begin to identify with you and copy your saner behavior.

We often feel more convinced by good examples than by other teaching methods. When someone tells us to buy a certain stock, or to shop at a particular store, we tend to have more confidence in the advice if we find that person investing in this stock or shopping at that store. Similarly, if you remain calm in the face of difficulties, behave in an adult manner in your vocational and social relations, and work things out in sensible instead of irrational ways, "neurotics" will more likely have faith in your views than if you act childishly and illogically. Perhaps the most effective of all methods of helping others, therefore, involves helping yourself with your own problems, and thereby setting a good example for them.

You can also help fairly troubled people by getting them actively interested in people and things outside themselves. For "neurotics," because of their extreme concern over approval by others, usually stay self-centered and not too interested in those around them. And others note this and in turn feel uninterested in them. This helps them to hate themselves more, especially when they realize they do not really care for anyone. Then they may feel ashamed of their inability to love.

Getting "neurotics" vitally interested in things and people outside themselves has several advantages. It distracts them from worries, gives them goals to live for, increases competency and success, and frequently provides them with other companions who serve as good models.

If, then, you can encourage troubled people to participate in outside ventures and get involved with others, you may appreciably help them. Don't, of course, push them into overly difficult tasks or into relationships with those likely to reject or damn them. But they often can make profitable contact with several others.

As noted in *A Guide to Rational Living*, a standard text on rational-emotive self-management that I wrote with Dr. Robert A. Harper, vitally absorbing interests (especially

creative ones) serve people best. If you can get emotionally
pained people occupied with writing rather than merely seeing plays, or with painting canvases rather than collecting
them, they will more easily absorb themselves in something
beside their neurotic whining.

The best help you can often give comes from inducing
"neurotics" to acquire a genuine interest in other people. Neurosis tends to take the form of a social disease, since it arises
when people devoutly believe that they *must* perform well
and win others' approval, that these others truly know and
loathe them for having inadequacies, and that they therefore
have to down themselves. One antidote to desperately need-
ing the approval of others comes with truly caring for those
others. Such loving will not only encourage others to love
in return; better still, it will often make the lover unfrantic
about whether they do or not.

Gaining the love of others indeed feels pleasant. But far
greater gains stem from loving actively and creatively yourself. We can see feeling loved as a passive occupation that
easily palls and bores. But loving involves a vitally absorbing,
active expression of yourself, a creative interacting between
your inner urgings and your environment. Loving, or creative
involvement in something outside yourself, moreover, helps
the problem of neurotic self-centeredness. For, by strong
concern with helping someone else grow and develop, you
may select a constructive, ongoing goal, have little time to
make yourself needlessly anxious, learn significant things
about the state of your own feelings, and have emotional experiences invaluable to your growth.

When I worked at a mental institution several years
ago, the director came to see me one day to discuss the problem of one of the Gray Ladies, or volunteer helpers, attached
to the institution. This woman acted in a high-strung, obvi-

ously disturbed way and the director had misgivings about taking her on. But he finally accepted her because she got along so well with some of the other Gray Ladies.

Once on the staff, she did her work well, and won the liking of all the inmates of the institution with whom she came into contact. There lay the trouble, the director said: she did so much for these inmates, to the extent of corresponding with them long after they left the institution, that some of the professional staff wondered if she established unhealthy relationships with them.

I could not see any great harm resulting from these relationships—but thought they might lead to some good, since the woman and the inmates both desired warm emotional attachments. I recommended, therefore, that the institution let her remain a member of the volunteer group.

Fortunately, I guessed right. Not only did the woman remain one of the best volunteer workers, but she gained so much by devoting herself to helping others that she felt considerably less disturbed. Although she at first experienced self-hatred, she gained so much vitality and enjoyment that almost everyone began to notice and comment on her improvement.

After a few more months, she did so well that, at the director's suggestion, she began to think of making a career of social work. In spite of the fact that she was forty-five years of age, she returned to school and obtained a social work degree. Although she never obtained any direct treatment, the indirect psychotherapy she obtained through her active interest in others helped her overcome some of her own serious problems.

If you encourage "neurotics" to develop an interest in others, you may thereby do them a good turn. But this may prove difficult, for their horror of rejection may prevent them from building relationships with others. In such cases you

[handwritten margin note: Ways to help neurotics to develop interest in others]

can help to break down their emotional blocks in several ways.

To make sure that they meet new and interesting people, introduce them to some of your own friends, take them to parties and gatherings, or get them to join social groups. Speak favorably of the people they may meet until they want to meet them. *[handwritten margin note: meet intrstg people]*

Help troubled people to get along better with others by showing that these people do not bar but often welcome friendship. Reveal that other people have problems too, and may therefore act rejectingly. Show them that others can display interest in them and provide valuable contacts. *[handwritten margin note: others want friends]*

Discourage flagging interest when troubled people suffer temporary setbacks in a relationship. Explain why particular individuals may not show enthusiasm and what can help build it. Indicate how they can learn not to take the negative attitudes of others too seriously. If you push them to develop companionable habits, in time their friendships may catch fire and grow, in spite of some setbacks. *[handwritten margin note: not taking neg attitudes of others too seriously]*

In several important ways, then, you can help disturbed persons to initiate and maintain intimate contacts with others, and thereby fulfill themselves. And, in so doing, you may succeed in inducing them to build affectionate relations with others that will truly minimize their neurotic self-centeredness.

You can also turn to one additional resource—getting neurotic friends or relatives to seek professional help. Disturbed people do not easily welcome help, and frequently construct important barriers against it. Even when they recognize the depth of their neuroses, they frequently feel so far gone, so hopeless, that they can't do anything about the situation. Despite all urging, they will not even try to get better. In such instances they can well use intensive psychotherapy.

To complicate matters still more, you may not easily overcome "neurotics'" refusal to accept therapy. They often will contend that professional help costs too much. Or say they have no time for it. Or point out that they know someone who has not benefited from it. Or admit they have fears of feeling psychologically torn apart and not knowing how to put themselves back together again. How, then, can you help reluctant "neurotics" to accept psychotherapy? Not by nagging! Explaining the virtues of psychotherapy and affirming your own belief in it may hardly help. Keeping after them may not achieve the desired result.

First convince them you want to help but have less ability than a competent therapist.

Also, if possible, introduce them to people who have had therapy and have felt helped by it. Or, if you know a good therapist socially, you can arrange for them to meet this individual so that they can see what a representative of the profession looks and sounds like.

Introduce those you want to help to sophisticated, educated people who realize the value of psychotherapy. If disturbed individuals only know relatively uneducated, defensive individuals—many of whom themselves have run from therapy—they will keep hearing the old bromide that only "crazy" people go for treatment. Try to show them that we can hardly label most therapy clients as "crazy," but more accurately describe them as people who have some serious problems. If you have had some therapy yourself, you may find it good to tell your neurotic friends about it and show them how you benefited from it. If one of them then shows interest, you may sometimes find it advisable to see a therapist first and explain your friend's problems, especially regarding reluctance to undertake treatment. You may thus prepare the therapist to overcome your friend's doubts and help him or her enter a full-scale therapeutic relationship.

Occasionally, you can half-trick someone into starting

108

therapy, particularly someone who really would like to have professional treatment but just will not endeavor to take the first step. Under these conditions you may use a ruse to get him or her into a therapist's office, if just for a single visit. Some of my own clients, for example, ostensibly see me first for the purpose of discussing someone else's problem—that of a wife, sister, parent, or child. In this manner they find out something about me, see if they think I can help them, and decide to begin a therapeutic relationship.

I had an experience of this kind when I saw a man whose wife had, according to his story, serious emotional problems but would not consider getting therapy. The husband and I discussed how we might possibly get his wife to see me; but whatever suggestions I offered he always discounted, fearing that they did not have sufficient subtlety, that his wife would see through them, and that she would absolutely refuse to come.

Finally, I suggested that he tell his wife that he worried about their seven-year-old daughter, whose behavior was something of a problem, that he himself couldn't give me too accurate a picture of her trouble, and that I would like to see the wife to discuss the daughter's difficulties.

As he predicted, the wife immediately made an appointment to discuss the daughter with me. But she had no sooner entered my office than she began talking about her own difficulties, especially those with her husband. Within fifteen minutes she had fully agreed that she herself could use treatment. By the time our first session ended, we had set up a schedule of future visits. When the husband learned of the results of my talk with his wife, he felt so astounded that he thought I had hypnotized her to win her over. Actually, I had done nothing but listen sympathetically to her complaints and show her that with regular psychotherapy she might find one way to get to the root of her disturbance.

This does not mean that people who fight off therapy

routinely need trickery to get them into it. Generally, such a method will do little good, because unless they want help, they usually won't accept it. But innumerable "neurotics," instead of solidly opposing therapy, feel ambivalent about it: they both want it and fear it. Many of these, after having some contact with a competent psychologist, easily manage to prolong that contact.

Can those who do not want therapy sometimes accept it with good results? Surprisingly, yes—sometimes. I have had clients sent to me by the courts after they had committed some offense. Although at first they came only because a judge forced them to come, later they developed into willing and eager clients and made considerable progress.

I have also had clients who came for only one reason: insistence by their husbands or wives. Most of them proved difficult and many left therapy after a few sessions, with little accomplished. But some of them, to my own surprise, went through an initial period of resistance and then settled down as hard-working clients.

As a last resort, when no other tactic will work, you may find it desirable to give neurotic friends or relatives a clear-cut ultimatum: that unless they accept professional aid, you will no longer help or perhaps even associate with them. Normally, this procedure won't work, but in a few cases it will.

On the whole, helping a "neurotic," or helping him or her get help, has distinct difficulties. But if you really care for and want to help a disturbed person overcome emotional problems, you can find this one of the most rewarding tasks you will ever undertake. By all means give a neurotic friend or relative a chance. You have little to lose, and often considerable to gain.

110

6

How to Live with a Person Who Remains Neurotic

Virtually all "neurotics" can improve—*if* they will get help and work hard for their own improvement. But many of them, for one reason or another, will not try to overcome their disturbances.

Sometimes they feel too old and tired to make the effort. Sometimes they will not do anything now, although they may hope to do something in the future. Sometimes the "neurotic" process has gone so far that they have little incentive to change. Sometimes they have beaten themselves down so thoroughly that they have little confidence left with which to fight for a change. Sometimes they fear any change, including getting better. Sometimes they can adjust moderately well to their disturbances and do not want to change.

Perhaps all "neurotics" can get better, but many of them will not. Even intensive psychotherapy will not produce good results, since they may resist using its teachings.

Suppose you live with a fairly disturbed individual who

simply will not accept help from you or anyone else. This could mean that your mate, a parent, or partner with whom you may have good reason for maintaining intimate contact stubbornly insists on remaining neurotic. How, under these conditions, can you live with this individual without making yourself upset? Let us examine some of the important techniques you can use.

First, fully, unequivocally accept the fact that disturbed people act in a peculiar, often obnoxious manner. I have chosen the words *fully* and *unequivocally* very carefully.

This may seem an unimportant point. But, no! "Of course," people tell me, "I know that So-and-So acts neurotically. I've known it for years. Naturally I make allowances for his disturbance."

Untrue! These people *think* they know So-and-So behaves neurotically; they *vaguely* know it. Actually and profoundly, however, they do not. And that makes all the difference in the world—the difference between vaguely acknowledging neurosis and *truly* knowing it.

Consider an example. One of my friends went with a woman for two years, kept telling me of her disturbed behavior, but then married her anyway because he wanted an interesting, intellectually alive companion. A few weeks after the marriage, he came to me and complained bitterly: "She doesn't do a thing. She doesn't read, she doesn't want to discuss anything interesting, she doesn't want to go visiting. She just sits on her behind all day and does nothing. How can I live with a woman like that?"

"But what do you expect," I asked, "from a 'neurotic'?"

"Oh, I see her neurosis, but—" And off he went into another tirade.

This man, however, did not *fully* see his wife's disturbance. If he had, he would have expected her to act in disturbed ways: to do exactly the kind of things she did.

Obviously he expected nothing of the sort and felt shocked when she acted neurotically. He said he unequivocally saw her neurosis. He thought he saw it. But no! It still took me a while to convince him of her true state and to help him *really* view her as neurotic.

Watch it! If you want to live peacefully with disturbed people, expect them to act neurotically. If you expect them to act perfectly sanely, rationally, and normally, what does that expectation show about *your* rationality? For you will then keep having your hopes fruitlessly raised—then dashed. No one, I trust, expects an infant to act like a grown-up, a professor like a Bowery bum. Why, then, should you expect a "neurotic" to act like a well-adjusted, mature individual?

Let us go over this once again—for you will probably find it *the* most important rule for living comfortably with "neurotics." You'd better *unreservedly* accept them as troubled, and expect them to act accordingly. Don't demand that they seem stable, sane, rational, logical, well-behaved, sober, mature, reliable, steady, hard-working, or anything else you may expect (and often fail to find) in non-"neurotics." Sometimes, especially for short periods, they may behave in a completely consistent, sound manner. But don't fool yourself. "Neurotics" will not keep this up indefinitely. If they could and would, we would not call them "neurotic"! Not accepting people with their disturbances amounts to blaming them for having them. And this helps them to act even more disturbed. For neurosis largely springs from people's internalizing and turning against themselves the criticism of others.

You may condemn troubled people directly or indirectly. Indirect blame may show itself in your distress. Thus, if you feel upset about your associates' behavior, they may see by your manner, if not by your words, that you think it "awful" or "terrible" for them to act the way they do. Sensing this, disturbed individuals often make themselves more neurotic.

We may attribute much of today's misery to so many "neurotics' " behaving in a typically disturbed manner, and to so many others' utterly refusing to accept them with this behavior. If only all of us—neurotic and normal—would realistically accept the fact that "neurotics" act neurotically, we would automatically feel less awful and experience less chaos when people act "wrongly."

All right! So Jones gets drunk every night and raises noisy hell. So Smith snubs us on the street. So Mrs. Henry spies on her neighbor's activities. What can we expect "neurotics" like Jones, Smith, and Mrs. Henry to do—behave soberly, nicely, and trustingly? We might just as well expect black to look white or a thief to root for law and order.

In accepting "neurotics" don't *personalize* their behavior toward you. Naturally, as a result of their disturbances, they will sometimes act negatively. But, as often as not, they treat you just as they routinely treat most other people, and, frequently, just as they treat themselves. They may seem, by their actions, vicious or stupid. Actually, they merely, because of neurosis, drive themselves to do vicious or stupid things.

Even when "neurotics" deliberately go out of their way to harm someone, we'd better not assume that they personally have something against that individual. At bottom, they remain personally against themselves and feel driven by self-hatred to hate others. Panic-stricken people, when caught in a fire, will ruthlessly knock down others to escape. But this does not mean that they hate these others or wish them harm. Similarly, "neurotics" frequently feel indifferent, sometimes even friendly, to a person even while, stricken with panic, they push that person out of their way. They don't necessarily *want* to do so; but feel forced to act antagonistically.

You can establish much better relationships with disturbed individuals if you learn to accept them and their acts with real knowledge about how and why they commit such

114

acts. If you refrain from personalizing, and try instead to see disturbed people in their own tragic light, you can greatly help them.

Let me give an illustration I frequently give my clients. Suppose you live with a neurotic male who compulsively gets up every morning at 3:00 A.M. and starts beating a set of kettledrums. This habit, to say the least, disrupts your sleep, and you want to do something about it. What can you do?

First, accept the fact that this person's drum-beating habits stem from his disturbance. Most probably, he doesn't beat the drums because he hates you, plots your death by physical exhaustion, or anything like that. He just has an "irrepressible" urge that he gives in to. Accept the fact that he has this urge. Don't make yourself angry. Remember that, in a way, this drum-beating harms him more than you. It constitutes *his* neurosis. Don't personalize it. Tell yourself, truthfully, that you suffer because of his disturbance—but you suffer because he acts neurotically, not necessarily against you.

So keep cool. Things seem bad enough at 3:00 A.M. without your trying to raise your own blood pressure and to commit murder. Keep telling yourself, over and over, if necessary, that your friend has emotional problems. Really convince yourself of this. And, because you convince yourself, remain calm—or, better, calmly determined to change things. *Then* you can best face the question of what to do about the situation.

The best thing, very frankly, might well involve one of you—you or this "neurotic's"—moving. If you find that you cannot easily survive under the existing conditions, by all means arrange to part company with your neurotic friend. Don't anger yourself at him. Don't blame him for having his disturbance. But determinedly, self-protectively, arrange for one of you to vacate the premises.

Suppose, however, this nocturnal drum-beater has a close relationship to you, and you won't bring yourself to live apart from him. Your next best move might include your re-arranging your living conditions so that you suffer little inconvenience from his symptoms. You can, for example, insist that he get a night job, so that he can beat the drums only during the day—when you, perhaps, work. Or see that he pays to have his room soundproofed. Or make some other arrangement that will let him keep his neurosis while you keep your sleep. In any event, remain determined and undisturbed, so that you can more effectively control the obnoxious, crazy situation.

To pursue the problem, suppose that you cannot stop your friend from beating his drums in the middle of the night and, for some reason, you don't want to change your living arrangements. You will then find it more important than ever to understand his neurosis and refuse to anger yourself about it. His keeping you awake nights seems bad enough. You make it much worse and keep yourself still more awake by hating him.

Accept his neurosis and its inconveniences. Convince yourself vigorously that he cannot easily help acting the way he does. Show yourself that the penalty (yours and his) for his neurosis means that you will continue to live under poor conditions until he changes, unless you manage to contain his neurosis or you get away from him.

Tell yourself that you could have things much worse. Instead of beating drums, he might beat you. Or he might beat the drums all night instead of merely for an hour or two. Or he might develop different but worse neurotic symptoms. So, if you choose to keep living with this disturbed person, by all means stop pitying yourself and telling yourself that unfairness *shouldn't* exist. You have, because of his neurosis, bad problems. But, really, *that* bad? And will making

116

yourself angry about them make things any better? On the contrary, worse!

Remain calm and determined. Accept your friend's neurosis for what it represents—an emotional disturbance. Don't try to fool yourself that you find it good and beneficial. But, at the same time, don't exaggerate its horrors. Accept it fully, realistically. Then, at least, you'll increase the possibility of your eventually doing something about it.

You can accept fully, and avoid getting unnecessarily perturbed by, the neuroses of your intimate by employing every bit of understanding of his disturbance that you may acquire. If you truly understand "neurotics" and keep reminding yourself *why* they act as they do, you will find it almost impossible to make yourself needlessly miserable over their behavior.

Another illustration I often give my clients: Suppose you walk down the street and a female friend leans out of a window and starts calling you all kinds of evil names. Would you feel badly? Normally, you would.

But if this same friend leans out of the window of a mental hospital and calls you exactly the same names, would you *then* feel as badly? Hardly!

Why? Why in the one instance would you make yourself vulnerable and in the other not? Because, obviously, you forgive the friend who leans out of the mental hospital. You *understand* that she has serious problems and that her name-calling results from disturbance rather than from her estimate of you or from anything you may have done. You tell yourself, in this latter instance, "Poor woman! She has lots of troubles, and therefore acts this way. When she improves, she probably won't call me those names."

The more you understand that people have neuroses and that their condition explains their actions, the less you will upset yourself about their behavior. By utilizing your understanding of disturbance, you make allowances for their annoying acts and feel less upset about it. Instead of building it up in your mind, as you would otherwise tend to do, you unconsciously start toning it down. You even feel intrigued, at times, with figuring out just *why* friends act in some particular neurotic manner. And, feeling intrigued, you do not damn them or down yourself.

Understanding breeds peace of mind. Primitive people who understood little about nature probably terrified themselves about things like eclipses, thunderstorms, and forest fires. We, because we understand these phenomena better, horrify ourselves less about them. Similarly, if you do not understand why "neurotics" act in a certain manner, you will feel perplexed and anxious about their behavior. But if you do understand the whys of such behavior, you will feel less perplexed. Even when you do not like neurotic behavior, greater understanding helps you feel calm about facing it.

You'd best learn as much about neurosis as possible and *use* this knowledge by reminding yourself: "I have some neurotic friends. They act this way because of their disturbances—for which they remain somewhat responsible, but not damnable. Let me, therefore, not take their neuroses too seriously nor deem them personally directed against me. Let me see if I can clearly understand some of their underlying feelings. Then, even if I can't help them, I will feel more comfortable myself."

When, for the moment, troubled people refuse to get help and continue to act in peculiar ways, some degree of emotional withdrawal may serve as the best way you can live comfortably with them.

Take the case of one of my clients, a nineteen-year-old male, a victim of agitated depression. Although he seemed bright, well-behaved, and talented, his parents criticized him severely. Members of a small sect, they felt that he should—

yes, should—live strictly in accordance with the ideals of this sect, which differed completely from the ideals of his friends. They expected him to have virtually no social life, to devote himself to politico-economic study, and to refrain from sex. He wanted to go out with females and to socialize with his male friends.

Because he followed his own bents, his parents criticized him more severely, called him a bum and a loafer, labeled him as immoral, and predicted he would never amount to anything. I saw both parents and tried to persuade them to moderate their criticism. To no avail. As soon as they realized I didn't favor their particular ideals, they began to think *me* a bum and a loafer, and concluded that I could not possibly help them and their son.

Since the son behaved more depressed by the day and could have ended in a mental hospital, I encouraged him to withdraw emotionally from his parents. I tried, at first, to get him to understand their disturbances, and to realize that their criticism stemmed from their own feelings of inadequacy. I helped inure him to their criticism: to predict, in advance, what they would say when he came home from a party or dance, and to avoid feeling upset about it. I showed him how they thought they did their best for him; but how, because of their own neuroses, they actually tried to get him to do everything *they* wanted, without really considering *his* desires, goals, and ideals.

Gradually, he pulled away emotionally from his parents. He lost his dependency on them; cared less what they thought of his behavior; understood their disturbances. The same disagreements and arguments continued at home, but now they did not affect him—he no longer took them seriously. Finally, when he felt undisturbed by anything his parents said, he got a job and moved out of the house. He saw his folks regularly and got along with them better than be-

119

fore. He even loved them in a quiet manner. But their pronounced influence on him had vanished, and he began, for the first time, to live his own life instead of mainly rebelling against the kind of life they wanted him to lead.

You may justifiably withdraw emotionally from people you love—your parents, for instance—in order to live more peacefully yourself. For if you love a "neurotic" unreservedly and devotedly, you take your emotional life in your hands. You can feel many kinds and degrees of love: mature love and immature love; romantic and calmer love; possessive and permissive love. If you love a "neurotic" in a mature, quiet, permissive manner, you will have more power to help that person and to maintain a healthier relationship with him or her.

Consider still another of my cases. The daughter, in this instance, felt great ambivalence toward her father: one day she hated him wildly, and the next day felt devoted to him. He behaved psychotically and had received treatment in several mental hospitals, but had never improved for more than a few weeks at a time. He would try to upset his daughter by telling her that she had cruelly sent him back to the hospital, and that if she really loved him she would take him to live with her and her family. I could see that if the daughter kept reacting badly to such emotional pressure, she would emerge as a prime candidate for a mental hospital herself.

I mainly helped the daughter to stop affecting herself about her father's charges. I got her for the first time fully to accept his disturbance, to see that she played no part in creating it, and to realize how foolishly she acted when she bowed to him or made herself guilty for not giving in.

As she gradually realized this, and made herself less upset, she changed remarkably. She acted more efficiently; she felt warmer to her children; her relations with her husband improved; and for the first time in many years she began to enjoy life. When her father called, she listened to him patiently, but did not take seriously anything he said. When he took turns for the worse, she felt prepared. When he returned to the mental hospital, she did not feel guilty or unduly upset. She fully understood his serious disturbance and that, since he did not permit her to help, she could do little for him.

You, too, can act this way, withdraw emotionally when involved with people who continually have problems. Understanding such people and refraining from condemning them, you still better not let them suck you in. Love a disturbed person—yes, but in a toned-down, cautious manner. Don't utterly sacrifice yourself, nor try to ape Florence Nightingale!

In other words, don't let neurotic or psychotic associates exploit your feelings. Keep some emotional distance from them and retain perspective in your attachments to them. Though charming, brilliant people, as a result of their neurotic limitations they generally have impoverished love relationships. They can give you just so much, because of their self-preoccupation. If you give without reservation, they frequently won't return your love in kind.

If, however, you find "neurotics" you love changeable, fine! If they will work at overcoming disturbance and at giving more love, by all means give generously to help them. But if they give up hope and refuse flatly to try to work to get better, beware! Out of self-protection, withdraw some of your attention, or, if necessary, break off the entire relationship.

Usually you won't find this more drastic action necessary. Even serious "neurotics," as a rule, have some capacity for warm relationships, and you can have limited love involvements with them. But recognize these limitations; don't delude yourself that they love deeply. Unless you relish unrequited love, care somewhat reservedly for disturbed people.

And if your relationships get too bad, wisely make a strategic retreat. Think of your own skin, for a neurotic intimate may have little regard for it.

Sometimes you cannot, emotionally or literally, get away from people with severely "neurotic" behavior. What can you do to live comfortably with them?

Acquire a more realistic, more stoical philosophy of life. You can use your head, as well as your heart, to overcome virtually any difficulty—including those that arise in attempting to live with "neurotics."

A rational, realistic philosophy of life includes several sane assumptions. First, the world has great difficulties and injustices—but you don't have to whine or make yourself furious about them. This in no sense implies that when things don't go the way you want them to go, you should not try to change them. Of course, try! But when you find things unchangeable—as on many occasions you will—don't wail or upset yourself about this.

Many so-called adults demand that the world work the way that they want it to work. They think it owes them a living. They insist that when things go wrong *no* justice or goodness exists. Mature adults think differently. They know we don't have the best of all possible worlds, but have much unfairness and injustice. They realize that more agreeable ways *can* occur. But they do not command that they *must*. In fact, wise people avoid almost all *musts*.

When you have a rational attitude, you make living your main purpose: experiencing, seeing, doing, feeling, existing. You try to make the most of your seventy-odd years by living them to the hilt; discovering as many vitally interesting things as possible; taking risks in order to gain certain pleasures; making clear-cut goals and plans and working to achieve them.

If you want to help make the world a little bit better than

when you came into it, great! You can choose to work for a "better" or "more peaceful" or "more just" world, in which you and other humans can live more happily, less neurotically.

But you'd better not equate working for a lovelier world with depressing yourself because it does not presently exist. The existing world, which we inherited and keep, has many obnoxious qualities—and many money-grubbers, tyrants, "psychopaths," and "neurotics." And quite likely it will have them for some time to come.

Moreover, aside from the current unsatisfactory state of the world, humans have great imperfections. They act more ignorantly, inefficiently, and nervously than they usually care to admit. They take considerable time to unlearn bad habits and learn better ones. They forget things easily. They inappropriately make themselves both overemotional and defensively underemotional. They have innumerable diseases and ailments. They frequently addict themselves to health-destroying habits. And these basic human limitations seem to go on forever.

Take, therefore, a realistic attitude! Don't necessarily *like* the world but *accept* its reality. If you don't like things, try to change them. If you can't change them now, stop whining and keep your eye on later. Don't give up living because life has hassles. Stop commanding that goodness *has to* exist.

As the philosopher Epictetus pointed out some two thousand years ago, we have practically no control over the activities of others. Why, then, *must* we control them?

If you live with "neurotics," think realistically. Don't, as we have stressed repeatedly, expect them to behave other than neurotically. And don't keep telling yourself "How awful that they act that way!" So your neurotic associates behave unfairly, unjustly. Who said that they *have to* act fairly? What law of the universe states that justice *must* exist? You certainly need not *like* their behavior. But hadn't you better, often, gracefully *lump* it?

You probably can't control disturbed people but you *can* control your own *reactions* to them. Not that you can completely avoid feeling annoyed when they do things you abhor. But you can work on your feeling of annoyance and tone it down, make it more bearable. You can expect an annoying event, for instance, and tell yourself it will probably happen. You can ask yourself how annoying you really find it. You can eliminate your upsettedness *about* feeling annoyed. Thus, you can accept the fact that "neurotics" *do* frustrate you and that you *do* dislike frustration. You can thereby reduce some of the annoyance you cause yourself. You can cut down on *surplus* annoyance. Don't spend too much effort trying to change "neurotics" who annoy you. Instead, change your own attitudes toward them.

You can reduce most annoyances by taking a rational or realistic attitude. Most such annoyances, when analyzed, consist of mere verbalizations, a matter of words. You bother yourself because someone calls you an evil name or otherwise expresses disapproval. Actually, however, the words or expressions don't hurt—for how can a word, in itself, hurt?—but your attitudes toward them can. If you *think* name-calling or rejection disastrous or horrible, you make it so. If you start thinking differently—realizing that mere words or expressions cannot hurt, you minimize verbal vulnerability and do away with much of your unhappiness.

As for the other kinds of annoyances in life, the actual physical ones—such as the painful sound of the drums at 3:00 A.M. or the real hurt of a blow on the head—you can also reduce these by taking realistic attitudes. You can sanely acknowledge that you cannot avoid all physical pain; that dwelling on it helps make it feel worse; that pain has certain advantages (helps to preserve life); and that, after taking measures to reduce it, you can avoid exaggerating physical harm. Other attitudes will almost certainly make you feel worse.

Moreover, you can often take steps to prevent the recurrence of physical pain. If you have headaches you can see a physician, learn the cause, and do something to eliminate them. If you have injuries, you can prevent repetition in the future by staying away from injurious situations.

The more balanced and determined you remain in the face of adversity, the more competently you can prevent its recurrence. If you upset yourself about headaches, you may actually avoid seeing a physician, for fear that he will tell you that you have some dread disease. If you make yourself enormously angry at someone who hurts you physically, you may not avoid that person but may actually seek him out, get into a real feud with him, and thus invite more blows. You can make physical ills worse, therefore, if you think crookedly about them and react to them in inappropriate ways.

You can employ several interesting methods of stubbornly refusing to upset yourself about adversity. For example, if you find yourself overreacting to neurotic behavior, you can ask yourself: "What difference does it really make? Because of Jim's neurosis, he keeps saying nasty things to me. Do they *really* hurt? Or do they hurt just because I *let* them hurt? Will he stop *liking* me because he says those things? Will I drop dead of a heart attack if I hear him say them? Will my boss fire me in the morning because of them? Of course not! Why, then, must I get so excited about what he says? Why give it an importance it really doesn't have?"

Using another approach, you might say to yourself: "Jim keeps making nasty statements about me. But what—at the very worst—can happen because of what he says? Perhaps he will no longer like me. Or he may turn others against me. Or I might lose my job because of his statements. Will it really spoil my whole life if any of these things happens? And even if I feel unhappy now, what effect will his words have ten years from now? Will I even remember this incident then? Probably not. So why need I make myself upset about it now?"

You can, as Epictetus demonstrated many centuries ago, use reason to eradicate virtually all emotional disturbances. But to employ these rational philosophies effectively, you'd better believe them! Telling yourself that an unpleasant event makes little difference now, nor will make any ten years from now, will not work if you really believe the opposite. Merely telling yourself will not suffice; you'd better thoroughly *convince yourself*. And you can. For you easily exaggerate the importance of what happens to you. If you consider its true importance, you will rarely seriously disturb yourself about it.

You can, of course, take to illogical extremes your questioning the importance of things! We all die, and though what happens today may well have little or no significance ten or a hundred years hence, we cannot accurately say that what happens today has *no* importance. If a neurotic associate, for example, hits you on the jaw, you will, at the very least, have a sore jaw. And that will seem quite important to you, if not to anyone else.

Don't tell yourself then that *nothing* has importance and that you should never feel concerned about anything. "Neurotics," in fact, typically convince themselves that they have no importance whatever, and that therefore whatever happens to them does not matter. To healthy individuals, what happens *does* matter. But not *too* much!

As usual, you can best solve the problem by taking an Aristotelian mean between two extremes—for instance, by adopting a philosophic attitude that enables you to live between the extremes of under- and over-exaggeration. Don't escalate the importance of things so that your life depends on them. But, also, don't convince yourself that nothing has any importance whatsoever. By all means find significance in whatever things you like. But if you cannot have them, don't believe the world has come to an end. You may well find it too bad to lose what you prefer, but not necessarily catastrophic.

See that you especially believe this when dealing with "neurotics." They often do inconvenient, annoying, shocking things. But, truly, will the world fall completely apart because of these neurotic acts? Or do you tend to make neurotic acts appear worse by overemphasizing their importance?

Try to stop harping upon the troubles "neurotics" cause and to accept them with their symptoms. Make every effort to think more philosophically about the annoyances they create. You can best live with troubled people by working to improve your own personality structure. Witness, in this respect, the work of professional therapists, who bring to therapy not only training and experience, but their own personality resources. They serve as good models for clients, refuse to enter into sick relationships with them as other weaker associates have done previously. And they can help give strength, because they preoccupy themselves so little with their own problems that they have sufficient time and energy to focus on those of others.

Good therapists rarely get disturbed by the antics of their clients in spite of the abuse they sometimes take. They accept name-calling, ingratitude, and condemnation and refuse to make themselves upset. They can do this partly because they think rationally and feel self-accepting (helped to some extent by their own training and therapy), and can therefore withstand abuse and have the willingness and ability to help the abuser.

Taking a lesson from the experience of psychotherapists, if you would best handle "neurotics," look into your own personality and see how *you* function. The better adjusted you behave, the greater the likelihood of your withstanding the annoyances that inevitably arise in relationships with disturbed individuals.

This does not mean you can simply say to yourself: "Now look here. You've just got to buck up and act non-neurotically yourself to live successfully with 'neurotics.' " Instead, take an inventory of your own traits and trends, try to understand as much as you can about neurosis in general and yourself in particular, and make some attempt to work through your disturbances.

To do a good job in this respect, you may benefit from some psychotherapy. Otherwise, you tend to remain too close to yourself to see objectively. You overlook your own neurotic trends. Or, when you find them, you feel inclined to rationalize or to work through them in a hazy, partial manner. Not that self-analysis has no value. As I and Dr. Robert A. Harper show in *A Guide to Rational Living,* you may find it extremely valuable. But for a thorough therapeutic job, you often can use the help of a well-trained, competent outside observer to assist you in your self-explorations and enable you to see many things you tend to keep out of awareness. For unconscious as well as conscious thoughts and feelings sustain your neurotic behavior. You often make yourself disturbed because you feel ashamed to face certain acts. (You irrationally think they prove you worthless.) And because you don't face them, you cannot easily change these unconscious defenses by yourself.

But with the help of a trained psychotherapist, you can reveal your unconscious thinking and understand yourself more fully. You can then unravel and work through your neurotic tendencies, and have more ability to help others.

A final word: "Neurotics," in our society, tragically abound. And this sad situation exists largely because humans in general and our culture in particular insist that we develop into champions, successes, and millionaires on the one hand, and angels, demigods, and saints on the other. But we can't have saintliness and have to fight like the devil to get it. And when we blame and damn ourselves for not achieving material success *and* sainthood neurosis almost inevitably results.

Our present society, then, at least escalates, if it does not fully produce, disturbances. Consequently, you will keep meeting many troubled people. As you do, remember this: "Neurotics" act neurotically. And you'd better not down them for having problems. They behave neurotically because they adopt irrational beliefs that lead to deep-seated feelings of inadequacy and hostility. They will tend to make themselves more disturbed if you make no allowances for their difficulties.

If *you* find it impossible to learn and apply these teachings about neurosis, you'd better suspect your own "neurotic" trends. If you can learn, as most probably you can, to apply them, you may well do yourself and others enormous benefit.

Will you accept this great challenge?

7

How to Live with Yourself though You Fail to Help a "Neurotic"

Let us suppose that you try all the things outlined in this book—you really, truly work at thinking and acting them through—and you miserably fail. The "neurotics" you try to help just won't listen to your wise words. Or they listen but intensely disagree. Or they agree that what you say and do makes great sense—but they still fail to follow your less neurotic ways and continue to behave abominably. Meaning: they treat you unfairly; they foolishly defeat themselves, while you suffer the consequences; they most sincerely promise you everything—and give you neurosis.

Naturally, if this occurs, you'll feel sorry. And frustrated! And thoroughly displeased! But will you—ah, will you?—also feel hurt? Depressed? Angry?

Maybe you won't. Maybe, applying the things you have begun to learn from this book about how others disturb themselves emotionally and how they don't have to do so, you will use rational-emotive principles on yourself, and stop yourself from this kind of upsetness.

Fine! But suppose you don't. Suppose, instead, you do let the behavior of your neurotic friends and relatives, and your own inability to help them change this behavior, get you down. What can you do then?

In the first edition of this book, I forgot to deal with this important problem. But now, with a hell of a lot of additional experience as a therapist under my belt, I see how often it arises and how infrequently it gets solved. For "neurotics" *do* avoid changing themselves—even when they go for therapy and spend a great deal of time and money supposedly trying to change. And people who attempt to help their disturbed associates *do*, in literally millions of cases, give up in disgust and break off intimate relationships with them—get a divorce, fire them, or refuse to see them again even when they have known them for years and perhaps brought them into this world.

It does happen; and so it may to you. If it does, and you find yourself failing completely with, giving up on, and perhaps even refusing to have anything more to do with "neurotics," how can you nicely continue to live with yourself, even though you have not succeeded in doing so with them? Let me summarize, to help you in this respect, some of the main techniques of rational-emotive therapy that you can apply to yourself if and when this happens.

The ABCs of Antiawfulizing. RET teaches people many things; but above all, it shows them how to stop awfulizing. Let us suppose that you keep doing this about your failure to succeed with your neurotic mother, mate, child, or friend. At point C, a Consequence, you feel ashamed and depressed, let us say, because your efforts with this neurotic individual have dismally failed. Point A (your Activating Experience) consists of noticing or acknowledging that you have failed and that this "neurotic" behaves as badly as, or even worse than, ever. Even though immediately after acknowledging your failure (at A), you feel depressed (at C), and even though you feel depressed when you think about this failure, *don't* assume that A causes or even directly leads to C.

Look for B—your Belief system! Ask yourself, first, "What rational Belief (rB) or sensible set of ideas do I probably tell myself, about A, in order to cause my reaction at C?" Answer: "Probably something like 'I don't like failing with my neurotic associate. I wish I had acted differently and had not failed. How annoying to put so much time and effort into this and still get such poor results! What a bother to have this person resist me so stubbornly!' "

Ask yourself, again: "If I stayed *only* with these kinds of evaluations of my failure with my neurotic associate, how would I probably feel about this failure, right now?" Answer: "Probably disappointed and annoyed. Maybe *very* disappointed and annoyed. But probably not much more than that."

Note, now: "But, honestly, my feeling, at point C, does *not* merely consist of disappointment and annoyance, nor even of *great* displeasure and irritation. If I face it, I feel pretty depressed—and probably also fairly angry—about what has happened. Therefore, if RET theory hits things correctly, I most probably keep strongly and persistently telling myself some highly irrational Beliefs (iBs) or idiotic ideas. Now what do I think those Beliefs might consist of?"

Answer: "I find it *awful* to have failed! I can't *stand* my acting so ineptly with my neurotic associate, and failing! I really *should* have worked more intelligently and persistently and have succeeded. And since I didn't do what I *should* have done, I clearly rate as a rotten person, a thorough incompetent!"

Admit that these irrational Beliefs (iBs) and *not* your failing with your neurotic associate (A) create your feelings of depression and shame (C). Then go on to Disputing (D) your irrational Beliefs, as follows:

(1) "What proof exists that life turns *awful* because I failed?" Answer: "None does! For *awful* means, first, highly disadvantageous or very inconvenient, which certainly could exist. Failing with this "neurotic" hardly brings me notable advantages or benefits! And it helps perpetuate the miserable state that I wanted to change. So it does seem obnoxious! But *awful* also means, in addition to highly disadvantageous, (a) that my failing proves 100 percent bad; (b) that it appears *more* than bad or at least 101 percent bad; and (c) that because it feels so bad, it *should* not, ought *not*, exist. Even the first of these propositions rings false (since 100 percent badness practically never exists in the universe); and the second and third propositions seem entirely magical. How can anything turn out *more than* or *worse than* obnoxious? It can't!"

(2) "Where have I any evidence that I can't *stand* my acting so ineptly with my neurotic associates and failing to help them?" Answer: "I don't have any such evidence! I'll never, of course, *like* behaving ineptly, if I did so act, and failing to help my neurotic friends or relatives. But I *can* stand what I don't like! In fact, I can stand *anything*, literally anything, that happens to me—as long as I remain alive. Even if someone tortured me to death, I could *stand* it—until, of course, I literally died. And failing to help a "neurotic" hardly seems as bad as getting tortured. So I'd better stop this nonsense about thinking I can't *bear* unpleasantries. Of course I can!"

(3) "How can I prove that I *should* have worked more intelligently and persistently and have succeeded with the

133

neurotics I have tried to help?" Answer: "I can't prove this. The statement 'I should have worked more intelligently' means two things: (a) 'It would have turned out more advantageously had I worked in this manner,' and (b) 'Therefore I *must* work more intelligently.' Although the first of these statements seems eminently sane and provable, how can I ever get evidence for the absolutistic *must* in the second statement? Clearly, I can't get such evidence. Indeed, if because something has advantages for me I *must* do it well, that law of the universe would *force me* to do advantageous things well. Clearly, however, I do many of them poorly. And clearly, none of these absolutistic *musts* exist."

(4) "What about my proposition, 'Since I didn't do what I *should* have done, I clearly rate as a rotten person, a thorough incompetent!'?" Answer: "Well, what about it? Clearly, it makes no sense. First of all, I have just seen that I can find no reason why I should have, must have, done well. Secondly, how could any rotten *people* exist? A rotten *person* would have to *always* and *only* act rottenly—which seems both unlikely and unprovable. And such a person, with a rotten-to-the-core *essence* would presumably get damned, by some all-powerful force in the universe, for having this essence. But does this seem likely—that some superhuman force spies on all of us humans, notices how rottenly we at times act, concludes that we rate as rotten *people,* and forever after devil-ifies us and damns us to perdition? Highly unlikely! And utterly unprovable. Moreover, if I believe that I rate as *thoroughly* incompetent, for making this mistake in trying to help my neurotic associate, how does that belief encourage me to act more competently in the future and make myself more helpful to some of the other 'neurotics' I know? It does nothing but help me *sabotage* my future behavior!"

In using the ABCs of RET in this manner, you can

quickly, in literally a few minutes, undo your awfulizing, at point B, about how you have failed to help your neurotic associate, at point B; and wind up with a new philosophy, or Effect (point E): "Well, I certainly feel sorry that I failed to help this person this time. But no matter how many times I fail, I shall keep trying: because it *only* remains unfortunate, and never awful and terrible if I fail, and I can always accept *myself* with my inept *behavior* and do my best to improve it in the future." When you believe this enough times, you have stopped your awfulizing in its tracks.

Rational-Emotive Imagery. You can use rational-emotive imagery (RET) created by Dr. Maxie C. Maultsby, Jr., and adapted by me, as follows: When you have failed with a neurotic associate and you tend to feel, let us say, depressed and self-downing for having failed, you imagine, as intensely as you can, this same thing happening again—and perhaps again and again. Thus, picture in your head your failing to help, say, your neurotic employer or supervisor. Fantasize this man remaining as nutty as ever: scolding you for minor errors, making undue demands on you, refusing to give you the kind of remuneration you really deserve, and acting most unpleasantly in spite of your best efforts to help him see the light and behave more sanely. As you fantasize this grim picture, you let yourself honestly feel depressed and defeated.

You then concentrate on your feelings in your gut and make yourself—yes, *make* yourself—feel only disappointed and annoyed. Not depressed. Not self-downing. Not angry. *Only* disappointed and annoyed. Don't think you can't do this, for you definitely can. You have real control over your feelings, no matter what conditions occur to you. So make yourself—again, *make* yourself—feel definitely bad about your employer's or supervisor's crummy, crazy behavior. But *not* depressed; *not* self-downing.

Keep at this until you succeed—if only briefly. Get at least a fleeting feeling of *mere* disappointment, mere sorrow, mere regret, mere annoyance. As soon as you have got this new feeling, notice what you have done in your head to create it. You probably have told yourself, to make yourself feel only sorrowful and disappointed, "The end of the world hasn't come! So he keeps scolding me for minor errors. Tough! So he makes undue demands. Too bad! So he won't pay me the kind of money I really deserve. What a pain in the neck! But I'll survive. I'll get by. I can still feel relatively happy and enjoy lots of other things in life, even though I may never enjoy working with him. Now, let me see what else I can do to make my life more enjoyable!"

Notice these things, you say to yourself. Notice your *new* philosophy, as you now feel only disappointed and not depressed and self-downing. See very clearly what you can think to make yourself feel regretful and annoyed but *not* terribly upset. Then, for at least ten minutes a day, do this same thing: fantasize some of the worst possible things happening, as your boss or supervisor remains very neurotic; and let yourself genuinely feel badly about this, but not depressed, not angry, not self-hating. Practice, for at least these ten minutes a day, feeling *appropriately* disappointed and annoyed but not *inappropriately* depressed and incensed. Practice, in other words, getting rid of your *demandingness* and replacing it with *desiring*. If you do this for at least ten minutes a day for several weeks, you will tend spontaneously and "automatically" to feel distinctly emotional, but *appropriately* emotional, if and when your boss or supervisor actually does treat you badly and unjustly.

If you do this kind of day-by-day rational-emotive imagery, great! If you don't, and you resolve to do it but don't actually carry it out (because you find it not only hard but "too" hard), look at the nonsense you keep telling yourself

and undo *those* foolish ideas. If necessary, use self-management or operant conditioning principles to get yourself to do
it regularly: reinforce yourself with something you find
highly pleasant (for example, eating, listening to music, talking to your friends, or reading only *after* you have done the
ten minutes REI for that day); and also, perhaps, penalize
yourself with something distinctly unpleasant (for example,
washing dishes for an hour, burning a twenty-dollar bill,
calling up someone you dislike speaking to, or eating some
unpleasant food) every day that you do not perform the REI.

Disputing Irrational Beliefs (DIBS). At the Institute for
Advanced Study in Rational Psychotherapy in New York
City, we have found that one of the exercises that people get
best results with in helping themselves change their self-
defeating ideas consists of Disputing Irrational Beliefs
(DIBS). You can practice this as follows:

Take any irrational Belief (iB) that you want to give up
and stop acting upon, such as the irrational Belief, "I must
succeed in helping my neurotic mate act much less neurotically," and write it down on a sheet of paper or record it on
a cassette tape recorder and then Dispute it with these questions, all of which you force yourself to think through very
carefully and to which you can write down or record the
answers:

1. WHAT IRRATIONAL BELIEF DO I WANT TO DISPUTE AND
SURRENDER?

Illustrative Answer: I must succeed in helping my neurotic mate act less neurotically.

2. CAN I PROVE THIS BELIEF TRUE?

Illustrative Answer: No, I don't think that I can.

3. WHAT EVIDENCE EXISTS OF THE FALSENESS OF THIS
BELIEF?

Illustrative Answer: (a) No law of the universe exists
that says that any "neurotic" that I care for *has* to improve

137

and behave less neurotically—although I would find it highly desirable if that person did!

(b) If this person proves unhelpable and continues to act just as neurotically as ever, it will certainly add to the inconveniences and hassles of my life, and will defeat his or her own happiness. But at worst, our lives will only prove very inconvenient. A hassle does not amount to a horror!

(c) If my mate continues to behave extremely neurotically and makes our lives together hardly worth continuing, we would again find that most inconvenient. But no evidence exists that my life and my mate's life *must* not turn out exceptionally troublesome.

(d) Other people live together, one or both of whom behave very neurotically, and somehow they manage to get along and even remain reasonably happy. If some of them can do so, there certainly seems ground for believing that my mate and I could do likewise.

(e) My demand that my neurotic mate act less neurotically amounts to an absolutistic *must*; and as far as I can see, *no* such absolutes exist, or at least can get factually substantiated, in the universe. If my mate *must* change and act less neurotically, then he or she *would* automatically change in that direction. Clearly, nothing of this kind keeps happening!

(f) In spite of the fact that my mate acts neurotically, and has continued to do so for years, we *do* have some enjoyable times together, *have* loved each other considerably, and *do* often get along well. Obviously, therefore, he or she doesn't *have to* act less neurotically for us to remain together and experience some degree of happiness.

(g) I would certainly act more efficiently and receive more enjoyment myself if I could help my mate act better. But that doesn't prove that I *have* to do so, nor that I rate as a total incompetent or failure if I fail to do so. It only proves my fallibility—which seems pretty obvious, anyway!

4. DOES ANY EVIDENCE EXIST OF THE TRUTH OF THIS BE-LIEF?

Illustrative Answer: No, not that I can see. Considerable evidence exists that if I did help my neurotic mate act less neurotically we both would get better results and lead a more enjoyable life. But that still doesn't prove that either or both of us *have to* improve and receive these favorable results. No matter how much anything *would prove better* that never means that *it must occur.* The main proposition that I can really substantiate about my mate's neurosis and my helping him or her change amounts to: "How desirable!" and not "How necessary!" I do not *need* what I *want.* Unless I foolishly *think* I do!

5. WHAT WORSE THINGS COULD ACTUALLY HAPPEN IF I DON'T GET WHAT I THINK I MUST (OR DO GET WHAT I THINK I MUSTN'T)?

Illustrative Answer: If my mate never acts less neurotically and I fail completely to help him or her do so,

(a) I would fail to get all the satisfactions I would like to get from living with him or her.

(b) I would receive, as would he or she, a good many extra inconveniences and annoyances.

(c) We might decide that we no longer find it worth living together and might break up our relationship.

(d) Other people, such as our family members, might suffer or get highly inconvenienced by our living together unhappily or deciding to part.

(e) Other people might down us and consider us pretty worthless for not getting along well together or dealing properly with my mate's disturbance—and that would prove distinctly annoying and unpleasant.

(f) I might go off and get involved with another mate who might prove just as neurotic, even more so, than my present partner; and that would seem really obnoxious!

(g) Various other kinds of misfortunes, unpleasant-nesses, and deprivations might occur, or continue to tran-spire, in my life. But none of these need I define as *awful, terrible,* or *unbearable.* At the very worst, they would remain problems and hassles—never *horrors* or *terrors.* Unless I foolishly *make them* so!

6. WHAT GOOD THINGS COULD I MAKE HAPPEN IF I DON'T GET WHAT I THINK I MUST (OR DO GET WHAT I THINK I MUSTN'T)?

Illustrative Answer: I can think of at least a few good things that might occur or I could make occur:

(a) If I find it impossible to help this mate with his or her disturbance, I could devote more time and energy, and receive a good deal of enjoyment, trying to help other people who may feel more receptive to my helping efforts—such as my children, my friends, my other relatives.

(b) If, as seems highly implausible, I could help no one overcome his or her neurosis, I could devote my time and energy to many other enjoyable pursuits. I could decide that this kind of thing just doesn't prove my bent, but that hardly means that I couldn't find many other satisfactions in life.

(c) Even my *attempts* to help my mate and others with their neurotic behavior, however much these attempts might fail, can prove highly interesting and enjoyable to me. *Striv-ing* for a desirable goal, though I never actually achieve it, can give a great deal of substance, vital interest, and fasci-nating direction to my life.

(d) I could find it exceptionally challenging and enjoy-able to teach myself how to live happily—though perhaps not *as* happily as might otherwise prove the case—even though I keep failing to help my mate act less neurotically. After all, I can make my main goal in life *my* getting along reasonably well in this difficult world. And even though I can often fail to change the world, I can certainly keep working at changing *me,* so that I stubbornly refuse to feel miserable when it continues to exist crummily. *That* kind of challenge can always seem exhilarating to me—if I stop my childish whining about the unniceties and inequities of the universe!

Again, as in your use of rational-emotive imagery (REI), you can use the Disputing Irrational Beliefs (DIBS) method for at least ten minutes a day, for a period of several weeks at a time. Take one major irrational Belief, such as the one we have just illustrated (or "I must do well at all the important things I do" or "Things in life have to come easily and rewardingly to me," or some other self-defeating philosophy), and vigorously dispute it every single day (including weekends!) until you really start to disbelieve it and act differently in connection with it. And once again, you can use self-management principles, as explained above in the section on rational-emotive imagery, to help yourself actually work these ten or more minutes a day at DIBS.

Referenting. Rational-emotive imagery, as noted in the introduction to this new edition of *How to Live with a "Neurotic,"* overlaps with the principles of general semantics as originated by Alfred Korzybski. For the main idea of general semantics consists of the principle that humans naturally and easily overgeneralize and resort to partially meaningless higher-order abstractions, and that they tend to defeat themselves and behave rather "insanely" (to use a term that Korzybski employed) by this poor semantic usage. Several writers on general semantics, such as Wendell Johnson, have tried to apply its teachings to the field of emotional disturbance, but they have usually tended to employ somewhat impractical and (ironically!) overgeneralized techniques. Rational-emotive therapy has used, since its inception, methods that seem more efficient and productive than other semantic methods in this connection.

141

Joseph Danysh, a dedicated general semanticist, has devised a referenting method that goes beyond other techniques in helping people overcome some of their self-defeating habits—especially that of smoking cigarettes. I have built somewhat upon his referenting methods and have applied them to various other kinds of emotional problems. If you want to use them in connection with your failing to help one of your neurotic associates, and your putting yourself down for this kind of failure, you may do so as follows:

Suppose you have failed miserably to help, say, your neurotic son; and this son continues to act badly and to get into all kinds of needless difficulties, some of which make life quite troublesome for you. Your problem basically consists of changing the meaning, or referents, of the terms *failing* and *succeeding*, so that whenever you think of these terms in connection with your son's continued neurotic behavior, you will feel appropriately sorry, sad, regretful, displeased, and annoyed, but not inappropriately horrified, terrified, angry, and self-downing.

You start with the term *failing*, and ask yourself: "What do I normally mean when I think about failing with my son and when I feel horrified and self-deprecating about this failure?" If you honestly ask this question, you will probably come up with an answer like: "I mean (1) his never having any happiness in life; (2) a miserable sinking in my own stomach; (3) the horror of the injustice of it all, that *my* son should act this way when I've tried so hard to get him to act better; (4) the disgrace of myself and my wife for having failed so miserably to raise our son better; (5) my own thorough ineptitude for not realizing earlier in his life how disturbed my son behaved and for not trying much harder to help him change."

In other words, your meanings or referents for the phrase "I have failed with my son" tend to consist of a few exceptionally negative ideas and feelings, some of them very self-downing and self-defeating. Almost automatically, whenever you think of your son's continuing disturbance—which you will almost inevitably think of on many occasions as you witness or imagine his behavior—you referent the terms "failing" and "son's neurosis" only—yes, only—with these awfulizing ideas and feelings. By so doing, without your realizing it, you keep *practicing* thinking and feeling depressed, anxious, and self-hating about your failing with your son. You continually *make yourself* feel this way, with your one-sided, bigoted, semantic usage.

The problem: to make yourself feel differently when you think of exactly the same terms that you now make yourself feel upset about. You take the term *failing to help son with his neurosis* and you think of it, in your head, as having quotation marks around it, thus, "failing to help son with his neurosis." But putting in the quotation marks you remind yourself, according to general semantic principles, that the term has *many* meanings, in fact, *all kinds of meanings,* in addition to the few awfulizing ones that you keep giving to it. And then you look for, and actually write on a piece of paper if you wish, some of these other meanings.

For example, objectively speaking, you can show yourself that "failing to help son with his neurosis" means such things as: (1) observing that he acts neurotically; (2) feeling displeased, for him and yourself, because he acts that way; (3) doing your best to show him how he behaves; (4) trying to show him how he might think, feel, and act differently; (5) actually helping him to change a little; (6) observing that he still often acts self-defeatingly; (7) realizing that many other sons, some of whom had very sincere and hard-working parents, still behave very neurotically; (8) experiencing annoyances, but hardly any outright catastrophe, from your son's continuing poor behavior; (9) seeing that other people, such as your son's friends, somehow tolerate him with his neurosis; etc.

Moreover, you can actively look for the positive referents that exist in regard to your son's disturbance and "failing to help son with his neurosis." Such positive referents might include: (1) your really doing the best you can do in this regard, in spite of the difficult circumstances involved; (2) your learning, in the process of trying to help your son, some valuable facts about human disturbance; (3) the special closeness you may have achieved with your mate, because you have this difficult problem of trying to help your son; (4) your discovering how to help your other neurotic associates and relatives better, through the information you gathered from trying to help your son; (5) your managing to achieve a good measure of self-acceptance and happiness, in spite of your failing with your son; (6) the interesting challenge presented by this very difficult problem of trying to get your son to change his behavior; etc.

If, whenever you think of the phrase "failing to help son with his neurosis," you *force* yourself—yes, *force* yourself—to think of all the possible referents you can attach to this phrase, and not merely of the highly negative, self-defeating referents you now almost exclusively keep attaching to it, the inherent *meaning* of this phrase will change for you and you will actually *feel* differently about it. In fact, as Danysh correctly indicates, you will automatically and spontaneously, after forcefully doing this kind of wide-ranging referenting for a while, feel relatively sorry, indifferent, or even (at times) good about your failure to help your son rather than only feeling intensely horrified about it. And Danysh's point—and the evidence I have gathered with many disturbed people whom I have taught to use referenting—tends to substantiate the major premise of rational-emotive therapy: that, basically, you feel the way you think, and that if you drastically change your irrational and one-sided thinking about something that keeps going wrong in your life, you will significantly, and sometimes dramatically, change your neurotic feelings about it.

To continue with the technique of referenting: After you make yourself call to mind all kinds of objective and positive referents regarding the phrase "failing to help son with his neurosis," you can do the same thing, if you find this desirable, with other phrases leading to your upsetness about this failure. You can, for example, take the phrase "son's neurosis" and force yourself to see that it not only means such things as "horrible disturbance," "worst thing that could ever happen to a human," "inordinately unfair and awful," "indubitably my fault," but that it also means several objective referents, such as "behavior accompanied by certain negative results," "actions that commonly exist among humans," "feelings that flow from irrational ideas," and "unfortunate behavior that arises from hereditary and environmental influences." On the positive side, you can also force yourself to recognize that "son's neurosis" also has some good or fortunate referents, such as "idiosyncratic traits that some people find charming," "interesting handicaps that give my son something to occupy himself with for the rest of his life," "creative trends that my son (and I) may use for purposes of learning, growth, and self-development."

Again, by insisting that you keep calling to mind *many* or *virtually all* the referents or meanings of the term "son's neurosis," you can get yourself to a point where you never quite wax enthusiastic about his having this set of characteristics but where you at least fully *accept* his having them and stop *horribilizing* about this kind of disadvantage or handicap. In a similar manner, you can take any word or set of phrases that you devoutly believe, and that keeps causing you to have disturbed feelings or to behave in a self-defeating manner

145

and you can referent many *other* meanings, beliefs, or attitudes that you can legitimately—and sometimes much *more* legitimately—connect with this same word or set of phrases. By vigorously forcing yourself many times to referent the more objective and pleasant meanings of this term or this phrase, you will eventually see it more realistically and less magically. In a sense, you will then more accurately know what the word or phrase *means;* and you will unconsciously and semi-automatically *feel* this more accurate, less self-defeating meaning. For don't forget, in this connection, words and phrases have no "true," "absolute," or "sacred" meaning. They mean what we *want* them or *make* them mean. And we always have the power to change these meanings, even when we keep the identical words or phrases. General semantics and rational-emotive therapy both posit and teach this view. If you follow general semantics principles, you normally make yourself saner and more rational—more competent to accept and live with reality. And so, too, with RET!

Homework assignments. Rational-emotive therapy stresses thinking, emoting, and behavioral homework assignments to help you change your ineffectual and emotionally disturbed tendencies. If you feel terribly depressed or self-downing about the fact that you have tried to help a "neurotic," and you would minimize or eliminate this feeling, you can devise various assignments to help yourself in this respect. Cognitive assignments would include using techniques like anti-awfulizing and DIBS, which I have just outlined in this chapter. Emotive assignments would include rational-emotive imagery.

Behavioral homework assignments might include such activities as deliberately forcing yourself to try to help another "neurotic," no matter how badly you have just failed with a close associate you have not helped; remaining for the present in the company of a neurotic relative or friend, in-

stead of avoiding him or her completely, in order to get practice in accepting this person's disturbed behavior; accepting
a job under a boss or supervisor who you feel pretty sure will
treat you neurotically as you keep working with him or her;
taking a counseling or personnel position, where you have to
deal with neurotic people constantly; determinedly confront-
ing a neurotic associate, such as your disturbed mother-in-
law, instead of trying to avoid the issue and not indicate that
you consider her behavior inappropriate.

You can also use self-management principles to get yourself to do activity homework assignments that you give yourself and do not actually carry out. Thus, if you decide to keep
working with neurotic intimates, even though you have
failed with one or more other "neurotics" recently, and you
keep avoiding doing what you have decided to do, you can
reinforce or reward yourself every time you do carry out this
kind of assignment, and quickly and sometimes drastically
penalize yourself every time you do not. You can also, of
course, using general rational-emotive principles, ask yourself, "In what way would I find it awful if I did carry out this
assignment?" and show yourself that it would not prove
awful or horrible, but merely unpleasant and unfortunate, if
you did the assignment—and that it would most probably
turn out *more* unpleasant if you did not.

By using some of the RET methods just outlined, as well as
those that I have described in *A New Guide to Rational Living, Humanistic Psychotherapy: The Rational-Emotive Approach,* and other writings, you can fully accept yourself
with your failure to help any "neurotics" whom you have
tried to aid. You can stop putting yourself down no matter
how badly you may do and no matter who thinks poorly
of you for your inefficiencies. You can ultimately, if you
do this often and vigorously enough, get to the point
where you automatically and spontaneously like or abhor

what you *do* without liking or abhorring *you* (rating *yourself*) for doing it.

If and when you do this, you will feel more able than ever to help "neurotics"—and will serve, in fact, as an admirable model for them. For neurosis, again, largely stems from profound *must*urbation: from the disturbed individual's devoutly believing (1) "I *must* do well and get approved for doing so, or else I rate as a pretty worthless person," (2) "You *must* act considerately and justly toward me, or else you turn into a villain," and (3) "The world *must* provide me with what I want quickly and easily, or else it proves awful and horrible!" If you give up—and I mean give up a thousand times —your own irrational *musts*, including "I *must* help my neurotic associates, otherwise I amount to practically nothing," you will tend to have an easier time encouraging and inducing "neurotics" to give up theirs.

Let me ask once again: Will you accept this great challenge?

Selected Readings

Warning! You might well take contemporary writing in the field of personality theory, clinical psychology, psychoanalysis, and psychiatry with many reservations. These writings have far to go in regard to scientific, verified knowledge.

The field of psychotherapy, moreover, tends to have many schools that believe they know exactly what makes humans "neurotic" and what to do about curing them. Unfortunately, however, these schools rarely agree on many important questions and tend to contradict each other.

Try to take modern psychological writings, therefore, with due skepticism, and largely consider them brilliant hypotheses that have yet brought forth little indisputable evidence. Continue to seek proof of their statements by further reading and thinking.

With this in mind, and with the hope that the readers of this book will take all psychological theories with many grains of salt, and will think for themselves before they firmly adhere to any, I offer the following list of supplementary readings. You may order items preceded by an asterisk, as well as obtain a price list, from the Institute for Rational Living, 45 East 65th Street, New York, N.Y. 10021.

ADLER, ALFRED. *Superiority and Social Interest.* Edited by H. L. and R. R. Ansbacher. Evanston, Illinois: Northwestern University Press, 1964.

———. *Understanding Human Nature.* New York: Greenberg, 1972.

ALBERTI, R. E., AND EMMONS, M. L. *Your Perfect Right: A Guide to Assertive Behavior.* San Luis Obispo, Calif.: Impact, 1971.

ANSBACHER, ·H. L., AND ANSBACHER, R. R. *The Individual Psychology of Alfred Adler.* New York: Basic Books, 1956.

ARD, BEN N., JR. (ed.). *Counseling and Psychotherapy.* Palo Alto, Calif.: Science and Behavior Books, 1966.

——, AND ARD,' CONSTANCE C. (eds.). *Handbook of Marriage Counseling.* Palo Alto, Calif.: Science and Behavior Books, 1969.

BACH, GEORGE R., AND DEUTSCH, RONALD M. *Pairing.* New York: Avon, 1973.

——, AND WYDEN, PETER. *The Intimate Enemy.* New York: Avon, 1971.

BANNISTER, D., AND MAIR, J. M. M. *The Evaluation of Personal Constructs.* New York: Academic Press, 1968.

BARKSDALE, L. S. *Building Self-Esteem.* Los Angeles: Barksdale Foundation, 1974.

BECK, A. T. *Depression.* New York: Hoeber-Harper, 1967.

*BEDFORD, STEWART. *Instant Replay.* New York: Institute for Rational Living, 1974.

BONE, HARRY. "Two Proposed Alternatives to Psychoanalytic Interpreting." In Hammer, E. (ed.). *Use of Interpretation in Treatment.* New York: Grune & Stratton, 1968, 169–96.

[BOURLAND, D. DAVID.] "The Un-isness of Is." *Time,* May 23, 1969, 69.

BULL, N. "An Introduction to Attitude Psychology." *Journal of Clinical and Experimental Psychopathology,* 1960, 27, 147–56.

BURKHEAD, DAVID E. *The Reduction of Negative Affect in Human Subjects: A Laboratory Test of Rational-Emotive Therapy.* Ph.D. thesis, Western Michigan University, 1970.

BURTON, ARTHUR (ed.). *Operational Theories of Personality.* New York: Brunner/Mazel, 1974.

*CRIDDLE, WILLIAM D. "Guidelines for Challenging Irrational Beliefs." *Rational Living,* vol. 9, no. 1, Spring, 1974.

CURTIN, MARY E. (ed.). *Symposium on Love.* New York: Behavioral Publications, 1973. *Rational Living,* Spring, 1974. 9(1), 8–13.

DANYSH, JOSEPH. *Stop Without Quitting.* San Francisco: International Society of General Semantics, 1974.

DAVIES, RAYMOND L. *Relationship of Irrational Ideas to Emotional Disturbance.* M.Ed. thesis, University of Alberta, Spring, 1970.

150

DAVISON, GERALD C., AND NEALE, JOHN M. *Abnormal Psychology: An Experimental-Clinical Approach*. New York: Wiley, 1974.

DEWEY, JOHN. *Human Nature and Conduct*. New York: Modern Library, 1930.

DI LORETO, ADOLPH. *Comparative Psychotherapy*. Chicago: Aldine-Atherton, 1971.

DORSEY, JOHN M. *Illness or Allness*. Detroit: Wayne State University Press, 1965.

*ELLIS, ALBERT. *The Art and Science of Love*. New York: Lyle Stuart, 1960. Rev. ed., New York: Lyle Stuart and Bantam Books, 1969.

*———. "Cognitive Aspects of Abreactive Therapy." *Voices: The Art and Science of Psychotherapy*, 1974, 10(1), 48–56.

*———. "Emotional Education at the Living School." In Ohlsen, Merle M. (ed.). *Counseling Children in Groups*. New York: Holt, Rinehart and Winston, 1973, 79–94. Reprinted: New York: Institute for Rational Living, 1974.

*———. *Executive Leadership: A Rational Approach*. New York: Citadel Press, 1972.

*———. *Growth through Reason*. Palo Alto: Science and Behavior Books, 1971. Hollywood: Wilshire Books, 1974.

*———. *Healthy and Unhealthy Aggression*. New York: Institute for Rational Living, 1974.

*———. *How to Master Your Fear of Flying*. New York: Curtis Books, 1972.

———. *Humanistic Psychotherapy: The Rational-Emotive Approach*. New York: Julian Press, 1973. New York: McGraw-Hill Paperbacks, 1974.

*———. *Is Objectivism a Religion?* New York: Lyle Stuart, 1968.

*———. "Is Psychoanalysis Harmful?" *Psychiatric Opinion*, 1968, 5(1), 16–124. Also: New York: Institute for Rational Living, 1969.

*———. "My Philosophy of Psychotherapy." *Journal of Contemporary Psychotherapy*, 1973, 6(1), 13–18. Reprinted: New York: Institute for Rational Living, 1974.

*———. "The No Cop-Out Therapy." *Psychology Today*, July 1973, 7(2), 56–62. Reprinted: New York: Institute for Rational Living, 1973.

151

——. "Outcome of Employing Three Techniques of Psychotherapy." *Journal of Clinical Psychology*, 1957, 13, 344–50.

——. "Psychotherapy without Tears." In Burton, Arthur (ed.). *Twelve Therapists*. San Francisco: Jossey-Bass, 1972, 103–26.

*——. "Psychotherapy and the Value of a Human Being." In Davis, J. W. (ed.). *Value and Valuation: Essays in Honor of Robert S. Hartman*. Knoxville: University of Tennessee Press, 1972, 117–39. Reprinted: New York: Institute for Rational Living, 1972.

——. "Rational-Emotive Therapy." In Corsini, R. (ed.). *Current Psychotherapies*. Itasca, Illinois: Peacock, 1973, 167–206.

*——. "Rational-Emotive Therapy." In Hersher, Leonard (ed.). *Four Psychotherapies*. New York: Appleton-Century-Crofts, 1970, 47–83.

*——. *Reason and Emotion in Psychotherapy*. New York: Lyle Stuart, 1962.

*——. *The Sensuous Person: Critique and Corrections*. New York: Lyle Stuart, 1972. New York: New American Library, 1974.

*——. *Sex without Guilt*. New York: Lyle Stuart, 1958. Revised ed. Hollywood: Wilshire Books, 1970.

*——. *Suppressed: Seven Essays Publishers Dared Not Print*. Chicago: New Classics House, 1965.

*——, AND BUDD, KATHIE. *A Bibliography of Articles and Books on Rational-Emotive Therapy and Cognitive Behavior*. New York: Institute for Rational Living, 1975.

*——, AND GULLO, JOHN M. *Murder and Assassination*. New York: Lyle Stuart, 1972.

——, AND HARPER, ROBERT A. *Creative Marriage*. New York: Lyle Stuart, 1961. Hollywood: Wilshire Books, 1973 (new title: *A Guide to Successful Marriage*).

*——. *A New Guide to Rational Living*. Englewood Cliffs, N.J.: Prentice-Hall, 1961; Prentice-Hall, 1975; Hollywood: Wilshire Books, 1975.

*——, KRASNER, PAUL, AND WILSON, ROBERT ANTON. "Impolite Interview with Dr. Albert Ellis." *Realist*, 1960, No. 16, 9–11; 1960, No. 17, 7–12. Reprinted: New York: Institute for Rational Living, 1970.

*——, WOLFE, JANET L., AND MOSELEY, SANDRA. *How to Raise an*

Emotionally Healthy, Happy Child. Hollywood: Wilshire Books, 1972.

EPICTETUS. *The Works of Epictetus.* Boston: Little, Brown, 1899.

FRANK, JEROME D. *Persuasion and Healing.* Rev. ed. Baltimore: Johns Hopkins University Press, 1973.

FRANKL, VIKTOR E. *Man's Search for Meaning.* New York: Washington Square Press, 1966.

FREUD, SIGMUND. *Collected Papers.* New York: Collier Books, 1963.

*GARCIA, EDWARD, AND PELLEGRINI, NINA. *Homer the Homely Hound Dog.* New York: Institute for Rational Living, 1974.

GILLETTE, PAUL, AND HORNBECK, MARIE. *Depression: a Layman's Guide to the Symptoms and Cures.* New York: Outerbridge and Lazard, 1973.

GINOTT, HAIM G. *Between Parent and Child.* New York: Macmillan, 1965.

GLASSER, WILLIAM. *Reality Therapy.* New York: Harper, 1964.

GOLDFRIED, MARVIN R., AND MERBAUM, MICHAEL (eds.). *Behavior Change through Self-Control.* New York: Holt, Rinehart and Winston, 1973.

*GOODMAN, DAVID, AND MAULTSBY, MAXIE C., JR. *Emotional Well-Being through Rational Behavior Training.* Springfield, Illinois: Charles C. Thomas, 1974.

GREENWALD, HAROLD (ed.). *Active Psychotherapies.* New York: Atherton, 1967.

———. *Decision Therapy.* New York: Wyden, 1974.

*GROSSACK, MARTIN. *You Are Not Alone.* Boston: Marlborough, 1974.

HADAS, MOSES (ed.). *Essential Works of Stoicism.* New York: Bantam Books, 1962.

HARPER, ROBERT A. *The New Psychotherapies.* Englewood Cliffs, N.J.: Prentice-Hall, 1975.

———. *Psychoanalysis and Psychotherapy: 36 Systems.* Englewood Cliffs, N.J.: Prentice-Hall, 1959.

———, AND STOKES, WALTER S. *Forty-Five Levels to Sexual Understanding and Enjoyment.* Englewood Cliffs, N.J.: Prentice-Hall, 1973.

HARTMAN, ROBERT S. *The Measurement of Value.* Carbondale: Southern Illinois University Press, 1967.

*HAUCK, PAUL A. *Overcoming Depression*. Philadelphia: Westminster Press, 1973.

*———. *Overcoming Frustration and Anger*. Philadelphia: Westminster Press, 1974.

*———. *The Rational Management of Children*. New York: Libra, 1967.

———. *Reason in Pastoral Counseling*. Philadelphia: Westminster Press, 1972.

HAYAKAWA, S. I. *Language in Action*. New York: Harcourt, Brace and World, 1965.

HERZBERG, ALEXANDER. *Active Psychotherapy*. New York: Grune and Stratton, 1945.

HORNEY, KAREN. *Collected Writings*. New York: Norton, 1972.

HOXTER, A. LEE. *Irrational Beliefs and Self-Concept in Two Kinds of Behavior*. Ph.D. thesis, University of Alberta, 1967.

JOHNSON, WENDELL. *People in Quandaries*. New York: Harper, 1946.

JONES, RICHARD G. *A Factored Measure of Ellis' Irrational Belief System, with Personality and Maladjustment Correlates*. Ph.D. thesis, Texas Technological University, 1968.

JUNG, C. G. *The Practice of Psychotherapy*. New York: Pantheon, 1954.

KELLY, GEORGE. *Clinical Psychology and Personality*. New York: Wiley, 1969.

———. *The Psychology of Personal Constructs*. New York: Norton, 1955.

*KNAUS, WILLIAM. *Overcoming Procrastination*. New York: Institute for Rational Living, 1974.

*———. *Rational-Emotive Education: A Manual for Elementary School Teachers*. New York: Institute for Rational Living, 1974.

KORZYBSKI, ALFRED. *Science and Sanity*. Lancaster, Pa.: Lancaster Press, 1933.

KRANZLER, GERALD. *You Can Change How You Feel*. Eugene, Oregon: Author, 1974.

LAUGHRIDGE, STANLEY THEODORE. *A Test of Irrational Thinking as It Relates to Psychological Maladjustment*. Ph.D. thesis, University of Oregon, 1971.

*LAZARUS, ARNOLD A. *Behavior Therapy and Beyond*. New York: McGraw-Hill, 1971.

*LEMBO, JOHN M. *Help Yourself*. Niles, Illinois: Argus Communications, 1974.

LEWIS, W. C. *Why People Change*. New York: Holt, Rinehart and Winston, 1972.

LOW, ABRAHAM A. *Mental Health through Will-Training*. Boston: Christopher, 1950.

*MACDONALD, A. P., AND GAMES, RICHARD G. "Ellis' Irrational Values." *Rational Living*, 1972, 7(2), 25–28.

MCGILL, V. J. *Emotion and Reason*. Springfield, Illinois: Charles C. Thomas, 1954.

MAES, WAYNE R., AND HEIMANN, ROBERT A. *The Comparison of Three Approaches to the Reduction of Test Anxiety in High School Students*. Washington: Office of Education, 1970.

MARCUS AURELIUS. *The Thoughts of the Emperor Marcus Aurelius Antonius*. Boston: Little, Brown, 1900.

MASLOW, A. H. *Motivation and Personality*. 2nd ed. New York: Harper, 1970.

———. *Toward a Psychology of Being*. Princeton: Van Nostrand, 1962.

*MAULTSBY, MAXIE C., JR. *More Personal Happiness Through Rational Self-Counseling*. Lexington, Kentucky: Author, 1971.

*———. *Help Yourself to Happiness*. New York: Institute for Rational Living, 1975.

———. *How and Why You Can Naturally Control Your Emotions*. Lexington, Kentucky: Author, 1974.

*———. "Systematic Written Homework in Psychotherapy." *Rational Living*, 1971, 6(1), 16–23.

*———, AND HENDRICKS, ALLIE. *Five Cartoon Booklets Illustrating Basic Rational Behavior Therapy Concepts*. Lexington, Kentucky: Authors, 1974.

MAULTSBY, MAXIE C., JR., STIEFEL, LEANNA, AND BROSKY, LYNDA. "A Theory of Rational Behavioral Group Process." *Rational Living*, 1972, 7(1), 28–34.

MEEHL, PAUL E. *Psychologists' Opinions as to the Effect of Holding Five of Ellis' 'Irrational Ideas.'* Minneapolis: Research Laboratory of the Department of Psychiatry, University of Minnesota, 1966.

MEICHENBAUM, DONALD H. *Cognitive Behavior Modification*. Morristown, New Jersey: General Learning Press, 1974.

———. *Cognitive Factors in Behavior Modification: Modifying What Clients Say to Themselves.* Waterloo, Canada: University of Waterloo, 1971.

MERRILL, M. G. "There Are No Absolutes." *ART in Daily Living,* 1972, 1(4), 6–9.

MEYER, ADOLPH. *The Commonsense Psychiatry of Dr. Adolf Meyer.* New York: McGraw-Hill, 1948.

*MORRIS, KENNETH T., AND KANITZ, H. MIKE. *Rational-Emotive Therapy.* Boston: Houghton Mifflin, 1975.

MOSHER, DONALD. "Are Neurotics Victims of Their Emotions?" *ETC. A Review of General Semantics,* 1966, 23, 225–34.

PAUL, G. L. *Insight versus Desensitization in Psychotherapy.* Stanford: Stanford University Press, 1966.

PERLS, F. C. *Gestalt Therapy Verbatim.* Lafayette, Calif.: Real People Press, 1969.

PHILLIPS, E. LAKIN. *Psychotherapy.* Englewood Cliffs, N.J.: Prentice-Hall, 1956.

RADO, SANDOR. *Adaptational Psychodynamics: Motivation and Control.* New York: Science House, 1969.

RIMM, DAVID C., AND MASTERS, JOHN C. *Behavior Therapy.* New York: Academic Press, 1974.

ROGERS, C. R. *On Becoming a Person.* Boston: Houghton Mifflin, 1961.

ROKEACH, MILTON. *Beliefs, Attitudes and Values.* San Francisco: Jossey-Bass, 1968.

———. *The Nature of Human Values.* New York: Free Press, 1973.

RUSSELL, BERTRAND. *The Conquest of Happiness.* New York: Bantam, 1968.

RUSSELL, PHILIP. *An Empirical Test of Rational-Emotive Therapy.* M.A. thesis, University of Kentucky, Lexington, Kentucky, 1972.

———, AND BRANDSMA, JEFFREY M. "A Theoretical and Empirical Integration of the Rational-Emotive and Classical Conditioning Theories." *Journal of Consulting and Clinical Psychology,* 1974, 42, 389–97.

SCHACTER, STANLEY. *Emotion, Obesity, and Crime.* New York: Academic Press, 1971.

SHARMA, K. L. *A Rational Group Therapy Approach to Counseling Anxious Underachievers.* Ph.D. thesis, University of Alberta, 1970.

SHULMAN, LEE M., AND TAYLOR, JOAN K. *When to See a Psychologist.* Los Angeles: Nash, 1969.

TAFT, G. L. *A Study of the Relationships of Anxiety and Irrational Ideas.* Ph.D. thesis, University of Alberta, 1965.

THEISEN, J. CHARLES. *A Study of a Psychotherapist: Albert Ellis.* M.A. Thesis, United States International University, 1973.

THORNE, F. C. *Principles of Personality Counseling.* Brandon, Vermont: Journal of Clinical Psychology Press, 1950.

TILLICH, PAUL. *The Courage to Be.* New York: Oxford, 1953.

*TOSI, DONALD J. *Youth: Toward Personal Growth, a Rational-Emotive Approach.* Columbus, Ohio: Merrill Publishing Co., 1974.

TREXLER, LARRY D. *Rational-Emotive Therapy, Placebo, and No-Treatment Effects on Public-Speaking Anxiety.* Ph.D. thesis, Temple University, 1971.

VALINS, STUART. "Cognitive Effects of False Heart-Rate Feedback." *Journal of Personality and Social Psychology,* 1966, 4, 400–408.

——, AND RAY, ALICE A. "Effects of Cognitive Desensitization on Avoidance Behavior." *Journal of Personality and Social Psychology,* 1967, 7, 345–50.

VELTEN, EMMETT C. *The Induction of Elation and Depression through Reading.* Ph.D. thesis, University of Southern California, 1967.

WALLING, CONNIE. "An Argument against the Desirability of Theoretically Presupposing Calm Indifference in Undesirable Life Situations." *ART in Daily Living.* 1972, 1(2), 3.

WEEKES, CLAIRE. *Hope and Help for Your Nerves.* New York: Hawthorn, 1969.

——. *Peace from Nervous Suffering.* New York: Hawthorn, 1972.

WIENER, DANIEL N. *A Practical Guide to Psychotherapy.* New York: Harper and Row, 1968.

——, AND STIEPER, D. R. *Dimensions of Psychotherapy.* Chicago: Aldin, 1965.

WOLBERG, LEWIS R. *The Technique of Psychotherapy.* 2nd. ed. New York: Grune & Stratton, 1968.

WOLFE, JANET L. "How Integrative Is Integrity Therapy?" *Counseling Psychologist,* 1973, 3(2), 42–49.

WOLPE, JOSEPH. *Psychotherapy by Reciprocal Inhibition.* Stanford: Stanford University Press, 1958.

———, AND LAZARUS, ARNOLD. *Behavior Therapy Techniques*. New York and London: Pergamon Press, 1966.

*YOUNG, HOWARD S. *A Rational Counseling Primer*. New York: Institute for Rational Living, 1974.

ZIMBARDO, R. G. *The Cognitive Control of Motivation*. Chicago: Scott, Foresman, 1969.

ZINGLE, HARVEY W. *Therapy Approach to Counseling Underachievers*. Ph.D. thesis, University of Alberta, 1965.

Tape Recordings, Films, and Videotapes

ELLIS, ALBERT. *John Jones. Tape recorded interview with a male homosexual*. Philadelphia: American Academy of Psychotherapists Tape Library, 1964.

*———. *Rational-Emotive Psychotherapy*. Tape recording. New York: Institute for Rational Living, 1970.

*———. *Theory and Practice of Rational-Emotive Therapy*. Tape recording. New York: Institute for Rational Living, 1971.

*———. *Solving Emotional Problems*. Tape recording. New York: Institute for Rational Living, 1972.

*———. *A Demonstration with a Woman Fearful of Expressing Emotions*. Filmed demonstration. Washington: American Personnel and Guidance Association, 1973.

*———. *RET and Marriage and Family Counseling*. Tape recording. New York: Institute for Rational Living, 1973.

*———. *A Demonstration with an Elementary School Child*. Filmed demonstration. Washington: American Personnel and Guidance Association, 1973.

*———. *A Demonstration with a Young Divorced Woman*. Filmed demonstration. Washington: American Personnel and Guidance Association, 1973.

*———. *Rational-Emotive Psychotherapy*. Filmed interview with Dr. Thomas Allen. Washington: American Personnel and Guidance Association, 1973.

*———. *Rational-Emotive Psychotherapy Applied to Groups*. Filmed interview with Dr. Thomas Allen. Washington: American Personnel and Guidance Association, 1973.

*———. *Twenty-one Ways to Stop Worrying*. Tape recording. New York: Institute for Rational Living, 1973.

*———. *How to Stubbornly Refuse to Be Ashamed of Anything*. Tape recording. New York: Institute for Rational Living, 1973.

———. *Twenty-five Ways to Stop Downing Yourself*. Philadelphia: American Academy of Psychotherapists Tape Library, 1973.

———. *Recession and Depression: or, How Not to Let the Economy Get You Down*. Philadelphia: American Academy of Psychotherapists Tape Library, 1973.

*———. *Cognitive Behavior Therapy*. Tape recording. New York: Institute for Rational Living, 1974.

*———. *Rational Living in an Irrational World*. Tape recording. New York: Institute for Rational Living, 1974.

*———. *The Theory and Practice of Rational-Emotive Psychotherapy*. Videotape recording. New York: Institute for Rational Living, 1974.

*———. *Conquering the Dire Need for Love*. Tape recording. New York: Institute for Rational Living, 1975.

*———. *Demonstration with Young Woman with Problem of Loneliness*. Videotape. New York: Institute for Rational Living, 1975.

*———, AND WHOLEY, DENNIS. *Rational-Emotive Psychotherapy*. A tape recorded interview. New York: Institute for Rational Living, 1970.

HARPER, ROBERT A., AND ELLIS, ALBERT. *A tape recorded interview*. Philadelphia: American Academy of Psychotherapists and Division of Psychotherapy of the American Psychological Association Tape Library, 1974.

HENDERSON, JOHN; MURRAY, DAVID; ELLIS, ALBERT; CAUTELA, JOSEPH; AND SEIDENBERG, ROBERT. *Four Psychotherapies*. Tape recorded interviews with the same anxious male. Philadelphia: American Academy of Psychiatrists, 1971.

MAULTSBY, MAXIE C., JR. *Decreasing Prescription Suicides*. Tape recording. Lexington, Kentucky: Associated Rational Thinkers, 1974.

———. *A Rational Behavioral Approach to Irrational Fears and Insomnia*. Lexington, Kentucky: Associated Rational Thinkers, 1974.

*———. *Overcoming Irrational Fears: Rational Behavior Therapy*. Series of cassette tape recordings. Chicago: Instructional Dynamics, 1975.

*WOLFE, JANET. *Rational-Emotive Therapy and Women's Problems*. Tape recording. New York: Institute for Rational Living, 1974.